Critical Care Focus

Critical Care Focus series

Also available:

H F Galley (ed) Critical Care Focus 1: *Renal Failure*, 1999.

H F Galley (ed) Critical Care Focus 2: *Respiratory Failure*, 1999.

H F Galley (ed) Critical Care Focus 3: *Neurological Injury*, 2000.

H F Galley (ed) Critical Care Focus 4: *Endocrine Disturbance*, 2000.

H F Galley (ed) Critical Care Focus 5: *Antibiotic Resistance and Infection Control*, 2001.

Critical Care Focus

6: Cardiology in Critical Illness

EDITOR
DR HELEN F GALLEY
Lecturer in Anaesthesia and Intensive Care
University of Aberdeen

EDITORIAL BOARD
PROFESSOR NIGEL R WEBSTER
Professor of Anaesthesia and Intensive Care
University of Aberdeen

DR PAUL G P LAWLER
Clinical Director of Intensive Care
South Cleveland Hospital

DR NEIL SONI
Consultant in Anaesthesia and Intensive Care
Chelsea and Westminster Hospital

DR MERVYN SINGER
Reader in Intensive Care
University College Hospital, London

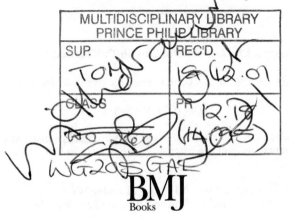

BMJ
Books

© BMJ Books 2001
BMJ Books is an imprint of the BMJ Publishing Group

First published in 2001
by BMJ Books, BMA House, Tavistock Square,
London WC1H 9JR

www.bmjbooks.com
www.ics.ac.uk

British Library Cataloguing in Publication Data

A catalogue record for this book is available from the British Library

ISBN 0-7279-1543-6

The chapters in this book are based on presentations given at the
spring meeting of the Intensive Care Society in Harrogate.

Typeset by FiSH Books London WC1
Printed and bound by Selwood Printing Ltd., West Sussex

Contents

Contributors

Stephen G Ball
British Heart Foundation Professor of Cardiovascular Studies, University of Leeds, Leeds.

Andrew J Bishop
Consultant Cardiologist, North Hampshire Hospital, Basingstoke.

David C Crossman
Professor of Cardiology, University of Sheffield, Sheffield.

Helen F Galley
Lecturer in Anaesthesia and Intensive Care, University of Aberdeen, Aberdeen.

John Hampton
Professor of Cardiology, University of Nottingham, Nottingham.

Max M Jonas
Consultant in Anaesthesia & Intensive Care, Southampton Hospitals Trust, Southampton.

Hugh Montgomery
Consultant in Cardiology, University College London, London.

Joseph E Parrillo
James B Herrick Professor of Medicine; Chief, Division of Cardiovascular Disease and Critical Care Medicine; Director, Section of Cardiology; and Medical Director, Rush Heart Institute at Rush-Presbyterian-St Luke's Medical Center, Chicago, USA. Editor-in-Chief of *Critical Care Medicine*.

Stephen Westaby
Consultant Surgeon, John Radcliffe Hospital, Oxford.

Preface to the Critical Care Focus series

The Critical Care Focus series aims to provide a snapshot of current thoughts and practice, by renowned experts. The complete series should provide a comprehensive guide for all health professionals on key issues in today's field of critical care. The volumes are deliberately concise and easy to read, designed to inform and provoke. Most chapters are produced from transcriptions of lectures at the Intensive Care Society meetings and represent the views of world leaders in their fields.

Helen F Galley

Introduction

Pathophysiology of heart failure

Stephen G Ball

Our understanding and management of acute heart failure has changed little in recent years, with a balance drawn between keeping inotropic support to a minimum, whilst ensuring adequate renal perfusion. In contrast, attitudes to the management of chronic heart failure have altered considerably. For the most part, heart failure is a result of myocardial damage from coronary artery disease, but nevertheless the underlying cause remains an important consideration in management strategies in the early stages, less so for end-stage heart failure. Considerable benefit has been shown following treatment with angiotensin converting enzyme inhibitors, and also from beta-adrenergic antagonists, after many years of avoiding their use in heart failure. The therapeutic benefit of these agents supports the concept that neurohormonal damage to the myocardium may be of more importance than haemodynamic factors in determining outcome. In this article the causes of chronic heart failure and current treatment issues are discussed.

Advances in the treatment of heart failure

John Hampton

An individual patient with heart failure can now be treated with a wide variety of drugs, all with a good evidence base to justify their use. The list includes digoxin, diuretics (including sprironolactone), angiotensin converting enzyme inhibitors and/or angiotensin receptor antagonists, and β-blockers. Many patients with heart failure will need some form of anticoagulant, and many – since they are on the whole elderly – will have other diseases that require other therapy. The clinical challenge is to select appropriate treatment for each individual patient: here guidelines can be singularly unhelpful.

Artificial hearts

Transcribed from a lecture given by Stephen Westaby and edited by Helen F Galley

Heart failure is a very significant problem and until recently there has not been an awful lot that a surgeon could offer to patients with end-stage heart failure. Although heart transplantation has been available since 1967, there is still a shortage of donors and some patients may not be suitable for transplantation. This article describes the different types of artificial hearts that are available and discusses the role for these in the management of heart failure.

How to use echocardiography

Andrew J Bishop

In normal cardiological practice, the echocardiogram is an indispensable tool in the diagnosis of haemodynamic disturbance. In the intensive care unit, where such disturbance is often much more critical, the echocardiogram can make crucial distinctions between the underlying causes of disease that require radically different approaches. The aim of this article is to persuade you that an echocardiogram in the intensive care unit can be useful and revealing. It concentrates on the use of echo to identify causes of haemodynamic compromise, and also addresses relevant technological advances.

Acute coronary syndromes

David C Crossman

The acute coronary syndromes encompass Q wave or transmural (full thickness) myocardial infarction and the non-Q wave myocardial infarct/unstable angina interface. The pathogenesis of these syndromes is believed to involve disruption of an atherosclerotic plaque in the majority of cases. Coronary plaque disruption appears to be either plaque fissure or superficial plaque erosion resulting in thrombus accumulation in the artery and hence the acute coronary syndrome. This article describes the therapeutic strategies available for this syndrome, which involves, for the main part, removal of the thrombus, prevention of further thrombus formation, and re-establishing adequate coronary blood flow. The emerging areas for treatment in the next 5–10 years will be lead primarily by changes in our improved understanding of acute coronary syndromes. Elucidation of events within the coronary vessel will almost certainly result in specific anti-inflammatory therapies for the vessel wall. Ongoing clinical trials of antibiotics in patients with unstable angina, following the suggestion that an infective agent may contribute to this condition, may also be fruitful.

Managing arrhythmias

Hugh Montgomery

Cardiac dysrrhythmia is common in the critically ill and is associated with impaired prognosis. The diagnosis of the abnormal rhythm and its management can often be difficult. This article aims to provide a clear and concise hands-on approach to the management of various types of arrhythmia in patients on the intensive care unit.

Estimation of cardiac output

Max M Jonas

The most important aspects of the cardiovascular system are blood pressure, volume and flow. All volume and flow measurements are indexed by expressing them in terms of body surface area, enabling comparison between individuals of different size and shape. Cardiac output is the ultimate expression of cardiovascular performance. It is the product of stroke volume and heart rate. Of course the magnitude of the stroke volume is determined by many other factors – preload, contractility, and afterload. Many people regard cardiac output as a measurement. However, cardiac output is not a measurement; a measurement is something that is obtained directly from a sensor. Cardiac output is, in fact, an indirect estimation, calculated from several other measurements, each of which is subjected to a range of specific errors. Quantitative estimation of cardiac output in most critically ill patients is made using the thermodilution method, but this technique has drawbacks, including expense and the requirement for a pulmonary artery catheter. Because of these problems, this method is restricted to patients in intensive care units. This article describes the methods currently available for the estimation of cardiac output, concentrating particularly on the lithium dilution technique as a safer alternative to thermodilution.

The heart and vasculature in sepsis and septic shock (Gilston Lecture)

Joseph E Parrillo

Septic shock is the commonest cause of death on intensive care units. Although sepsis usually results in low systemic vascular resistance, there is strong evidence for depressed myocardial function. In this article the incidence and pathogenesis of septic shock and the characteristic cardiovascular abnormalities, in addition to current therapeutic approaches, are described. It is clear that much of the pathophysiology of sepsis and the cardiovascular system remain incompletely understood. As the complicated mechanisms involved become clearer, physicians will be in a better position in terms of treating our patients, and soon we may be able to offer effective specific treatment for this very devastating disease.

1: Pathophysiology of heart failure

STEPHEN G BALL

Introduction

Our understanding and management of acute heart failure has changed little in recent years, with a balance drawn between keeping inotropic support to a minimum, whilst ensuring adequate renal perfusion. In contrast, attitudes to the management of chronic heart failure have altered considerably. For the most part, heart failure is a result of myocardial damage from coronary artery disease, but nevertheless the underlying cause remains an important consideration in management strategies in the early stages, less so for end-stage heart failure. Considerable benefit has been shown following treatment with angiotensin converting enzyme inhibitors, and also from beta-adrenergic antagonists, after many years of avoiding their use in heart failure. The therapeutic benefit of these agents supports the concept that neurohormonal damage to the myocardium may be of more importance than haemodynamic factors in determining outcome. In this article the causes of chronic heart failure and current treatment issues are discussed.

Causes of heart failure

It should be remembered that heart failure is not a diagnosis. There has to be an underlying cause for the heart failure (Box 1.1). For the majority of patients, this is undoubtedly ischaemic or coronary heart disease. Although severe hypertension *per se* may lead to the development of heart failure, particularly if the blood pressure rises relatively quickly such that the heart is not prepared for it, hypertension usually results in heart failure via underlying coronary artery disease. People with diabetes are particularly at risk of developing chronic heart failure, again as a consequence of ischaemic heart disease. Other causes, such as valvular disease and cardiomyopathy, or congenital abnormalities, are relatively uncommon in the community, although seen regularly in the hospital.

Box 1.1 Causes of heart failure

- Coronary/ischaemic heart disease
- Hypertension
- Diabetes
- Valvular disease
- Cardiomyopathy
- Congenital abnormalities

In a study published in the *Lancet* in 1997, McDonagh *et al.*[1] screened over 1400 men and women aged 25–74 living in the community in Glasgow, for impaired ventricular function. The prevalence of left ventricular (LV) systolic dysfunction, defined as a LV ejection fraction of 30% or less, was 2·9% overall. It increased with age and was higher in men. More than 80% of those with systolic dysfunction had evidence of ischaemic heart disease compared with 21% without systolic dysfunction. Hypertension was also more common in those with systolic dysfunction. These authors recommended the screening of groups at high risk for LV systolic dysfunction.

Physiology of chronic heart failure

Most patients with chronic heart failure have a normal cardiac output at rest but have limited cardiac reserve; they cannot increase their cardiac output adequately when necessary. In the past, therapy was directed towards increasing cardiac output using inotropes. Improvement, if any, would be temporary. Diuretics can also help. They lower filling pressure, and decrease pulmonary oedema, but concurrent shrinkage of circulating blood volume leads inevitably to oliguria and fatigue. When cardiac output falls, sympathetic activity is switched on, driving the heart but also causing vasoconstriction and raising blood pressure, thereby adding to its workload. The loss of output from the heart can be counteracted by increasing its filling pressure (Frank–Starling mechanism). Volume expansion of the circulation can be achieved through stimulation of the renin–angiotensin–aldosterone and arginine–vasopressin systems. Such correction of volume is appropriate if blood has been lost from the circulation. However, when the problem lies with the heart as a pump these corrective physiological responses are not helpful. Vasoconstriction makes the work of the heart harder, and sodium and water retention results in pulmonary oedema. It was realized then that the compensatory mechanisms were also causing problems for the heart itself. The circular consequences of the physiological compensatory mechanisms involved in heart failure are shown in Figure 1.1.

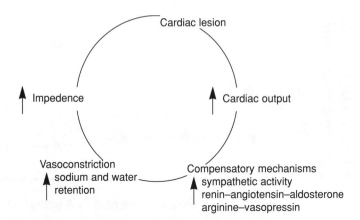

Figure 1.1 The cycle of compensatory mechanisms involved in the development of heart failure.

The underlying myocardial damage

When a myocardial infarction occurs the myocardium is deprived of its blood supply and the damaged ischaemic heart wall bulges out uselessly as the heart contracts. The undamaged remaining part of the ventricle contracts normally or with increased effort to compensate for the damaged area. With time the damaged area stretches and thins and fibrous tissue replaces what was once viable myocardium. The heart dilates and remaining viable myocardium hypertrophies. This process can be elegantly demonstrated using modern magnetic resonance imaging. Histological examination of damaged ischaemic hearts reveals that patchy areas of fibrosis develop even outside the infarct area. Myocardial cells are seen surrounded by collagen in the failing heart and in these areas apparently remote from ischaemic damage, fibres may be degraded and metalloproteinases reshape the surrounding matrix.[2] Myocytes become elongated and hypertrophied.

Gaudron *et al*[3] showed that almost a half of patients develop measurable LV dilatation within 4 weeks of myocardial infarction. Such dilatation is compensatory, restoring cardiac output and stroke index at rest and preserving exercise performance. However, of these, some 20% of patients develop progressive dilatation, which although compensatory initially, progresses to severe LV dysfunction (Figure 1.2).

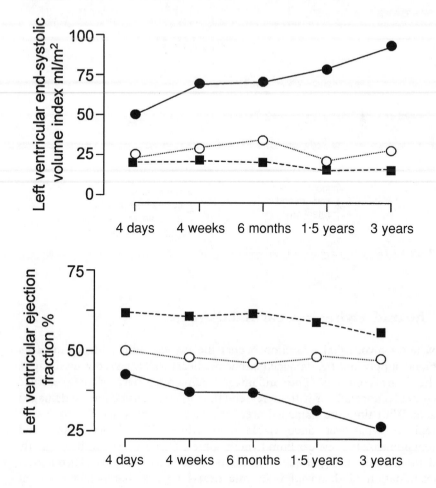

Figure 1.2 Course of left ventricular end systolic index and ejection fraction in patients with progressive (closed circles), limited (open circles) and no (closed squares) ventricular dilatation from 4 days to 3 years after myocardial infarction. Data reproduced with permission from Gaudron et al.[3]

Mechanisms of remodelling in heart failure

The processes driving this remodelling are interesting. The normal heart mass is provided mainly by myocardial cells, although in terms of number many more cells in the heart are fibroblasts. Cells have few options in terms of response to signals: they can function normally, divide or differentiate, hypertrophy, or undergo cell death either by apoptosis (programmed cell death), or by necrosis. Myocytes in the heart are terminally differentiated, and a number in the normal heart undergo apoptosis such that myocytes are also lost in an age-related non-inflammatory manner. Cardiac myocytes can also hypertrophy in part to compensate for any loss in number. In the presence of ischaemic damage necrosis may occur, providing a stimulus for fibroblast proliferation. Fibroblasts are very different from cardiac myocytes in that they can divide and synthesize large quantities of collagen leading to the observed fibrosis characteristic of ischaemic heart failure.

Two signals that have been shown to regulate cellular activity are the sympathetic and renin–angiotensin (RA) systems (Figure 1.3). The active mediator of the RA system is the octapeptide angiotensin II (Ang II), which is formed from the removal of the terminal two amino acids from angiotensin I (Ang I) by ACE. Angiotensin I is produced from its precursor, angiotensinogen, by the action of renin in the circulation, but also in tissues. In the heart Ang II can be formed in the absence of ACE; the most well characterized pathway is via chymase activity. Ang II acts on two types of receptors. The AT_1 receptor seems to be the key receptor causing vasoconstriction, release of aldosterone and also important growth effects. The role of the AT_2 receptor is less clear but it may have antiproliferative actions. The formation of Ang II can be blocked by ACE inhibitors, or its action at the receptor site by AT_1-blockers. There is a lot

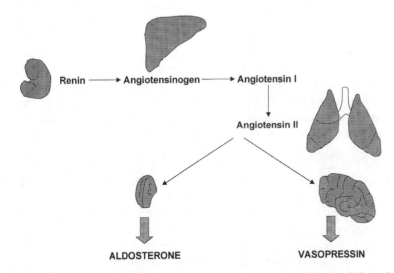

Renin ──────▶ Angiotensinogen ──────▶ Angiotensin I

Angiotensin II

ALDOSTERONE　　　　　　　　　　**VASOPRESSIN**

Figure 1.3 The renin–angiotensin–aldosterone system. Renin produced by the kidney cleaves angiotensinogen produced by the liver to angiotensin I, which in turn is cleaved by angiotensin converting enzyme in the lung to angiotensin II. Angiotensin II stimulates the secretion of vasopressin from the posterior pituitary and aldosterone from the adrenal cortex. Both angiotensin II and aldosterone act on the nephron to stimulate sodium ion reabsorption resulting in a decrease in sodium excretion. Renin production is increased in response to decreases in perfusion pressure, increased sympathetic nerve activity or decreases in sodium chloride delivery to the macula densa. Decreases in renin release occur when perfusion pressure increases, sympathetic nerve activity decreases, and sodium chloride delivery increases. In addition, atrial natriuretic peptide and angiotensin II switch off renin release.

of interest in whether there are important differences according to the mechanism of inhibition chosen.

Twenty years ago, in 1980, Sharpe et al[4] reported the effect of the ACE inhibitor captopril on haemodynamics in patients with severe chronic heart failure. Patients showed improvements in symptoms, exercise tolerance, and echocardiographic indices of LV size and function. More recently, the same group in Australia and New Zealand[5] reported beneficial ventricular remodelling in patients with heart failure from ischaemic heart disease after treatment with the β-adrenergic blocking drug, carvedilol. These studies demonstrate the importance of both the renin–angiotensin and the sympathetic nervous systems in the mechanism of ventricular dilatation in heart failure. Confirmation of the benefit from ACE inhibitors and the addition of β-adrenergic blockers has been seen in a series of major large studies.[6-8]

Although perhaps half of patients with ventricular dysfunction show progressive ventricular dilatation, eventually succumbing from chronic heart failure, many patients die suddenly and it was previously thought that these patients died from arrhythmias. There is no doubt that large areas of connective tissue and myocardial damage provide the substrate for severe arrhythmia, but many patients may have further myocardial infarctions. The causes of death in patients with heart failure are shown in Box 1.2. Both the β-blockers and the ACE inhibitors have now been shown to be able to prevent myocardial infarction, and this may be one of the mechanisms by which they are so effective in improving outcome in patients with heart failure.[9-11] Ideally, of course, we would like to be able to prevent *adverse* progressive myocardial fibrosis after infarct, although some fibrosis may be beneficial. An important approach is to prevent damage at the time of the initial coronary occlusion. Although thrombolytic therapy or angioplasty is essential to re-open vessels, and can achieve good reperfusion, opening the artery is not always a solution. Patency may be achieved too late and sometimes patent vessels opened by angioplasty can be observed to carry blood as a conduit, but have little effect on tissue perfusion (reviewed by Goldstein and Oz[12]).

There are factors other than the sympathetic nervous system and the renin–angiotensin system, which have important roles in what happens to the heart during heart failure. The sympathetic system remains incompletely understood since although β-blockers have been very effective, when the drug moxonidine was given to block sympathetic output centrally, this was not shown to benefit to outcome from heart failure (presented to the European Society of Clinical Cardiology, Barcelona 1999). There are other mediators (Box 1.3), including peptides such as endothelin, and cytokines tumour necrosis factor-alpha (TNFα), interleukin-1 (IL-1), and IL-6. Drugs such as pentofylline may provide benefit. Also, growth factors like transforming growth factor beta (TGFβ), have been implicated in the ventricular remodelling process. The problem with these mediators is knowing whether they are driving the process or whether they are just secondary.

Box 1.2 Causes and risk of death in chronic heart failure

- 50% unexpected
  - arrhythmia
  - myocardial infarction
  - pulmonary embolism
  - stroke
- 50% pump failure
  - repeat myocardial infarction
- Increased risk of dying
  - long duration of heart failure (50% dead within 5 years)
  - worse left ventricular function
  - symptoms of ventricular failure

Box 1.3 Other possible therapeutic targets in heart failure

- Blockade of sympathetic output centrally – monoxidine
- Endothelin antagonists
- Cytokine inhibition – TNFα, IL-1, IL-6 blockade, pentoxifylline
- Vasopeptidase inhibition
- Aspirin/warfarin

Conclusion

Heart failure occurs commonly after myocardial infarction. Ventricular remodelling and dilatation may progress from a compensatory phase to severe LV dysfunction. Sympathetic activity and the renin–angiotensin–aldosterone pathways, are involved and their adverse effects can be ameliorated in part through either β-blocking agents or ACE inhibition. An interesting question is whether the initial damage is the key determinant of outcome or whether further on-going ischaemic damage plays an equal role.

7

References

1 McDonagh TA, Morrison CE, Lawrence A, *et al*. Symptomatic and asymptomatic left-ventricular systolic dysfunction in an urban population. *Lancet* 1997;**350**:829–33.

2 Spinale FG, Coker ML, Bond BR, Zellner JL. Myocardial matrix degradation and metalloproteinase activation in the failing heart: a potential therapeutic target. *Cardiovasc Res* 2000;**46**:225–38.

3 Gaudron P, Eilles C, Kugler I, Ertl G. Progressive left ventricular dysfunction and remodeling after myocardial infarction. *Circulation* 1993;**87**:755–63.

4 Sharpe DN, Douglas JE, Coxon RJ, Long B. Low dose captopril in chronic heart failure: acute haemodynamic effects and long-term treatment. *Lancet* 1980;**2**:1154–7.

5 Doughty RN, Whalley GA, Gamble G, MacMahon S, Sharpe N. Left ventricular remodeling with carvedilol in patients with congestive heart failure due to ischemic heart disease. *J Am Coll Cardiol* 1997;**29**:1060–6.

6 Flather MD, Yusuf S, Kober L, *et al*. for the ACE-Inhibitor Myocardial Infarction Collaborative Group. Long-term ACE-inhibitor therapy in patients with heart failure or left-ventricular dysfunction: a systematic overview of data from individual patients. *Lancet* 2000;**355**:1575–81.

7 CIBIS-II Investigators and Committees. The Cardiac Insufficiency Bisoprolol Study II (CIBIS-II): a randomised trial. *Lancet* 1999;**353**:9–13.

8 MERIT-HF Study Group. Effect of metoprolol CR/XL in chronic heart failure: Metoprolol CR/XL Randomized Intervention Trial in Congestive Heart Failure (MEROT-HF). *Lancet* 1999;**353**:2001–7.

9 Ball SG, Hall AS. How ACE inhibitors reduce death from myocardial infarction: hypotheses from the Acute Infarction Ramipril study. *Br J Clin Pract* 1996;**84**(Suppl.):31–5.

10 Yusuf S, Peto R, Lewis J, Collins R, Sleight P. Beta blockade during and after myocardial infarction: an overview of the randomised trials. *Prog Cardiovasc Dis* 1985;**27**:335–71.

11 Yusuf S, Sleight P, Pogue, Bosch J, Davies R, Dagenais G. Effects of an angiotensin-converting-enzyme inhibitor, ramipril, on cardiovascular events in high-risk patients. The Heart Outcomes Preventions Evaluation Study Investigators. *NEJM* 2000;**342**:145–53.

12 Goldstein DJ, Oz MC. Current status and future directions of minimally invasive cardiac surgery. *Curr Opin Cardiol* 1999;**14**:419–25.

2: Advances in the treatment of heart failure

JOHN HAMPTON

Introduction

There is a now a large evidence base that supports the use of a wide variety drugs in the treatment of patients with heart failure (Box 2.1). Most of the trials that form this evidence base had as their endpoints the reduction of death or hospital admission; there are relatively few large and good trials that address the problem of symptomatic improvement.

Box 2.1 Drugs to be considered for the treatment of chronic heart failure

- Digitalis
- Diuretics
- Nitrates
- Other vasodilators
- ACE inhibitors/angiotensin receptor antagonists
- β-adrenergic blockers
- Inotropes
- Amiodarone

The management of acute left ventricular (LV) failure with diamorphine, intravenous diuretics and vasodilators such as intravenous nitrates has not changed for many years, and here mainly the treatment of chronic heart failure is discussed. When considering 'advances' in treatment based on clinical trials it is important always to bear in mind the fact that clinical trials in heart failure tend to include relatively young men who have no other diseases and who are not receiving other treatments. In the real world of heart failure the common patient is an elderly woman with multiple diseases who is receiving a variety of other treatments; the 'evidence base' for treating such patients may not be as secure as is often assumed.

The effective treatment of heart failure goes back 200 years to William Withering's introduction of digitalis, obtained from foxglove leaves. From his own observations he knew the sort of patient that digitalis helped – the typical one had cold and clammy skin and a feeble intermittent pulse. He did not know about acute LV failure, nor about atrial fibrillation, and certainly he had not considered the need for evidence-based practice, but he set off an argument about the efficacy of digoxin that was not solved until all of these aspects were understood. The way the place of digoxin was established provides an example for the introduction of all other treatment strategies in heart failure.

One of the first things that Withering recognized was that digitalis did not work in all forms of 'dropsy'. For example, it was ineffective – and indeed dangerous – in ovarian dropsy. We do not find this surprising, because we now know that ovarian dropsy is actually an ovarian cyst, and not a form of heart failure at all. He also knew that digitalis was ineffective when used for ascites from alcoholic cirrhosis, but many of his colleagues did not appreciate this; this led, in part, to the belief that digitalis was dangerous. What we now appreciate is that the cause of heart failure must be established before heart failure is treated: arrhythmias must be corrected, and problems that are amenable to surgery – valve disease, LV aneurysm – must be corrected. Heart failure as such is treated when a diagnosis of the cause has been made, and any primary treatment that is possible has at least been set in train.

One of the things we do not yet know is how many more causes of heart failure need specific treatment. For example, we do not know whether revascularization, either by percutaneous transluminal coronary angioplasty (PTCA) or coronary artery bypass grafting (CABG) is useful in the treatment of heart failure from coronary artery disease. When considering pharmacological 'advances', we have to remember that there are many basic questions still to be resolved, even though we have at our disposal an increasing number of effective drugs. With these caveats, however, we can consider the evidence for some of the drugs now in use.

Digoxin and other inotropes

When digoxin was the only effective treatment for heart failure, there was little need to test its efficacy. However, as other treatments became available – first the mercurial, then the thiazide, and the loop diuretics – the value of digoxin began to be questioned. In the United Kingdom particularly, there was a widely-held belief that its only value was in the control of the ventricular rate in patients with atrial fibrillation. The value of digoxin in patients with sinus rhythm was not established until the Digitalis Investigators Group (DIG) study was published in 1997[1] (Table 2.1). In this study digoxin or placebo were added to all other standard treatments in patients with heart failure, who were in sinus rhythm and who had a LV ejection fraction of 45% or less. The death rate over a 3-year follow-up period was 1181/3397 (34·9%) among the patients given digoxin, and 1194/3403 (35·1%) among those given placebo. This similarity in death rate in both treatment groups disguised the important fact that there were significantly fewer deaths from increasing heart failure in the digoxin group, but more deaths that were sudden or due to myocardial infarction. There were fewer hospital admissions in the digoxin group. Digoxin can therefore be seen to have a useful effect in reducing heart failure but no effect on overall mortality. The other important finding in this study – by no means unique – was the very high death rate among heart failure patients. The patients included were not especially ill – over half had symptoms in the New York Heart Association (NYHA) category 2 – and all these patients were already being treated with diuretics and angiotensin converting enzyme (ACE) inhibitors.

Table 2.1 Results of the DIG trial

	Placebo $n = 3899$	Digoxin $n = 3889$
Total deaths	1263	1274
Heart failure deaths	463	401
Hospitalizations for heart failure	1263	1274

Reproduced from: Digitalis Investigators Group. *NEJM* 1997;**336**:525–33.[1]

Apart from digoxin, all the drugs with a positive inotropic effect that have been tested in long-term trials have been shown to *increase* the mortality of heart failure patients. Despite the fact that such drugs improve symptoms, and despite some of them at least being valuable for short-term support in severely ill patients, such drugs clearly have no place in long-term management. These drugs include amrinone, milrinone, enoximone, flosequinan, and ibopamine.

Diuretics

Diuretics have for many years been the mainstay of heart failure treatment, and they still are. There are few, if any, trials that demonstrate their effect on symptoms, but most would argue that it is so obvious that trials are unnecessary. More worrying is the lack of trials investigating their effect on survival.

There have been no survival studies involving the thiazide or loop diuretics. The only important diuretic trial is that of spironolactone, the Randomized Aldactone Evaluation Study (RALES).[2] The patients included were those in NYHA categories 3 and 4 (i.e. they were severely ill) and they were all treated with digoxin, diuretics, and ACE inhibitors. Only a low dose – 25 mg or 50 mg daily – of spironolactone was used. Over a 2-year treatment period, spironolactone reduced mortality from 44% to 34%, and the hospitalization rate was also reduced (Table 2.2).

Table 2.2 Results of the RALES trial

	Placebo $n = 845$ (%)	Spironolactone $n = 832$ (%)
Deaths	44	34
Hospitalizations	91	81

Reproduced from: Pitt B, et al. NEJM 1999;341:7709–17.[2]

ACE inhibitors and angiotensin receptor antagonists

ACE inhibitors have been shown to improve the survival of patients with all degrees of heart failure, whether following a myocardial infarction or not, and also to prolong survival in patients with asymptomatic LV dysfunction and even those simply at high risk of developing heart disease.[3] ACE inhibitors do not totally block the conversion of angiotensin I to angiotensin II, so theoretically one might expect that a drug that blocks the angiotensin II receptor would be even more effective. Furthermore, some of the unwanted effects of ACE inhibitors – particular angioneurotic oedema and cough – may well be due to bradykinin, the effects of which are potentiated by ACE inhibitors. The appearance of a totally new class of drugs (the 'sartans'), which block the angiotensin receptors (there are several), thus caused considerable excitement.

The first heart failure trial involving a drug of this class (losartan) was called ELITE.[4] Seven hundred patients were included, and the aim was to compare the effects of losartan and captopril on renal function. As was expected, there were no differences between the two drugs in their effect on renal function, but an unexpected finding was a marked reduction in deaths, and particularly in sudden deaths, among the patients treated with losartan. Since this was a finding that was not a principal endpoint of the trial it had to be checked in a second study (ELITE II),[5] which was specifically designed to study the effect of losartan on mortality. In this study there was no significant difference in death rate among groups of patients treated with losartan or an ACE inhibitor.

Whether ELITE 2 has given us the final word on the efficacy of angiotensin receptor antagonists remains to be seen. It is possible that other drugs in this class, which have different effects on the different angiotensin receptors, may have different clinical effects. It is also possible that a combination of an angiotensin receptor antagonist and an ACE inhibitor may be more effective than either drug alone. Trials now in progress may answer these questions.

β-blockers

ACE inhibitors are effective in heart failure because they counteract the unwanted vasoconstriction caused by the activation of the renin–angiotensin system in heart failure. The autonomic system is also active in heart failure, with more vasoconstriction owing to both neural and hormonal effects, and it is logical that inhibition of the sympathetic axis would have benefits in the same way as inhibition of the renin–angiotensin system. One would, of course, have to expect unwanted effects, for it has always been recognized that β-blockers can precipitate heart failure.

A series of studies has now shown that if β-lockers can be tolerated by a patient in heart failure, survival is prolonged. The most convincing of these studies (CIBIS 2)[6] studied the effect of bisoprolol, which was given in addition to an ACE inhibitor. The starting dose was extremely low (one quarter of the smallest commercially available tablet) and the dose was increased very slowly, at monthly intervals, until the more usually dose of 10 mg daily was reached. Mortality was reduced from 17·3% in the placebo group to 11·8% in the patients given bisoprolol (Table 2.3).

Table 2.3 Results of the CIBIS II trial

	Placebo n = 1271 (%)	Digoxin n = 1322 (%)
Deaths	17·3	11·8
Hospitalizations	41	33

Reproduced from: *Lancet* 1999;**353**:9–13.[6]

This is probably a 'class effect' of β-blockers because similar benefits have been demonstrated by trials of carvedilol[7] and a slow-release form of metoprolol.[8] However, the difficulty of using β-blockers in heart failure must not be underestimated. Patients characteristically feel less well for the first few weeks of treatment, and many develop worse heart failure and treatment has to be abandoned – indeed, many patients simply will not take their tablets. However, if a patient with moderate heart failure can be established on a β-blocker, their outcome will undoubtedly be improved.

Conclusions

An individual patient with heart failure can now be treated with a wide variety of drugs, all with a good evidence base to justify their use. The list includes digoxin, diuretics (including spironolactone), ACE inhibitors and/or angiotensin receptor antagonists, and β-blockers. Many patients with heart failure will need some form of anticoagulant, and many – since they are, on the whole, elderly – will have other diseases that require other therapy. The clinical challenge is to select appropriate treatment for each individual patient; here guidelines can be singularly unhelpful.

References

1   Digitalis Investigators Group. The effect of digoxin on mortality and morbidity in patients with heart failure. *NEJM* 1997;**336**:525–33.
2   Pitt B, Zannad F, Remme WJ, *et al*. Effect of spironolactone on morbidity and mortality in patients with severe heart failure: RALES. *NEJM* 1999;**341**:7709–17.
3   Anonymous. Effects of ramipril on cardiovascular and microvascular outcomes in people with diabetes. Results of the HOPE study and microHOPE substudy. Heart Outcomes Prevalence Evaluation Investigators Group. *Lancet* 2000; **355**:253–9.
4   Pitt B, Segal R, Martinez FA, *et al*. Randomised trial of losartan versus captropil in patients over 65 with heart failure: ELITE study. *Lancet* 1997;**349**:747–52.
5   Pitt B, Poole-Wilson PA, Segal R, *et al*. Effect of losartan compared with captopril on mortality in patients with symptomatic heart failure: randomised trial (ELITE II). *Lancet* 2000;**355**:1582–7.
6   Anonymous. The cardiac insufficiency bisoprolol study II (CIBIS II): a randomised trial. *Lancet* 1999;**353**:9–13.
7   Packer M, Bristow MR, Cohn JN, *et al*, for the US Carvedilol Heart Failure Study Group. *NEJM* 1996;**334**:1349–55.
8   MERIT-HF Study Group. Effect of metoprolol CR/XL in chronic heart failure: Metoprolol CR/XL randomised intervention trial in congestive heart failure. *Lancet* 1999;**353**:2001–7.

3: Artificial hearts

transcribed from a lecture given by STEPHEN WESTABY
and edited by HELEN F GALLEY

Introduction

Heart failure is a very significant clinical problem and until recently there has not been much that a surgeon could offer to patients with end-stage heart failure. Although heart transplantation has been available since 1967, there is a shortage of donors and some patients may not be suitable for transplantation. This article will describe the different types of artificial heart that are available and discuss the role for these in the management of heart failure.

Surgical options in end-stage heart failure

There are some surgical options for some patients with end-stage heart failure, apart from transplantation.[1] Coronary bypass grafting alone will help patients with reversible ischaemia. Many patients with heart failure have mitral regurgitation, and it used to be thought that in these patients, if the mitral valves were repaired, the left ventricle would be unlikely to cope with the load. However, this is now known to be untrue and in particular in patients with dilated cardiac myopathy and grades III and IV mitral regurgitation, mitral valve repair is useful. Left ventricular (LV) aneurysm can be resected, and structured operations to remodel the failing left ventricle coupled with coronary bypass can also help. However, in patients with no reversal ischaemia and very large LV end-systolic volumes of more than 100 ml/M^2, right ventricular failure, pulmonary hypertension, and high central venous pressure, this is the stage where there is practically nothing conventional surgery can offer.

Transplantation

Although heart transplantation is available and may be a viable option for some patients, there are only about 280 transplants a year in the UK at the moment and there are hundreds of thousands of patients with heart failure. Box 3.1 shows heart transplant figures from Germany between 1997 and 1998. In this study 6000 patients with heart failure were initially investigated with a view to transplantation but only 1000 of those were referred and 500 were listed for transplant. Two hundred patients actually received a heart and 160 patients were alive after 1 year. These data reveal that survival out of this particular potential transplant group was only 2–3%.

Box 3.1 Heart transplantation and survival in Germany 1997–1998

- 6000 patients with heart failure
- 1000 patients referred for transplant
- 500 patients listed for transplant
- 200 transplanted
- 160 alive at 1 year
- 2–3% alive at 5 years

It has been suggested that xenotransplantation, i.e. pig organs, may be an option. In my opinion, such strategies are still as far away now as they were 10 years ago, and this is also the opinion of many transplant surgeons.

Artificial heart

It is clear that there is room for a different approach.[2] Chronic immunosuppression, allograft coronary disease and restricted availability of donor organs limit the scope of cardiac transplantation. The concept of replacing failing hearts with a mechanical device as a bridge to transplant has been accepted for a number of years. Indeed, the first artificial heart was developed in the 1950s; in those days the artificial organs actually looked like hearts. The patient's own heart was removed and was replaced with a pump that would mimic the functions of both the left and right sides of the heart. The only totally artificial heart that was used in a widespread manner for bridging until transplant was designed by Robert Jarvik – called the Jarvik 7. It is a pneumatic device, and mechanical heart valves determine the path of the blood. The process of filling, exiting and refilling is much like a normal human heart. Until very recently this is what was thought to be the best mechanism an artificial heart was thought to need. The first patient who received the Jarvik 7 was a dentist from Utah. However, the procedure was something of a disaster, since the patient's chest was unable to be closed at the end of the operation and then further surgery was needed to replace a failed mechanical valve.

Left ventricular assist devices

It was later realized that support of both sides of the heart was not required. Approximately 92% of patients with end-stage LV failure can manage on LV support alone with LV assist devices or LVAD. Such a device is manufactured by Novacor and there are many patients living out in the community in Germany, France and the United States with these devices implanted on a long-terms basis.[3-5] New technology means that these devices are powered electrically rather than the previous pneumatically driven devices. They provide an effective means to support the circulation, although there is a high incidence of infection, thromboembolism and stroke. These devices are used both for patients waiting for a transplant and for longer term ventricular support, and appear to be particularly useful when there is no other treatment option.[5] Neuroendocrine function is generally abnormal in patients with cardiac failure and a requirement for cardiac support. Use of an LVAD device has been shown to be associated with an improvement of neuroendocrine function.[6]

The success with the use of first generation LVAD devices that were designed 20 years ago, not only as a bridge to transplant but also for long-term mechanical circulatory support for 2, 3 and now 4 years, stimulated the evaluation of permanent artificial heart devices for patients who were not eligible for transplantation. Initially the Thermocardiosystems artificial heart was used. This device had a much lower thromboembolism rate than the Novacor devices. The first implant of the new electric version of this device was very successful. One patient, a man in his sixties, who was a diabetic and was not eligible for transplant received one of these devices. The function of his own left ventricle was very carefully studied using continuous echocardiography. Initial studies from the United States had suggested that, with chronic mechanical offloading, the patient's own heart function improved, and indeed this is what happened with this gentleman. His own heart got better – the artificial device had provided a bridge to recovery.

Bridge to recovery

This bridge to recovery concept came from earlier trials of bridge to transplant, where transplant surgeons found that mechanical offloading had resulted in myocardial recovery on both a cellular and molecular level.

17

This was shown by taking biopsies from the apex of the patient's heart when the artificial device was implanted, and then examining the heart again when it was removed for transplantation. The cellular hypertrophy observed consistently in heart failure was seen to improve, and the ventricle was able to remodel as it was offloaded. LV function recovers remarkably with chronic offloading. These findings supported the idea that patients with heart failure can be treated with artificial LVAD to rest their heart, leading to remodelling and recovery – the patient can then keep his own heart and the pump can be removed.

Although initial clinical experience with this is limited, it is certainly encouraging. The sustainability of the recovery remains unknown. We do not yet know what happens when the device is removed or whether the same pathological process results in heart failure at a later stage.

A couple of cases serve to illustrate the bridge to recovery concept. A 21-year-old girl was referred from an intensive care unit in London virtually moribund, on a balloon pump ventilator. She had viral myocarditis and, although this will often resolve with time, heart failure may result before recovery. The patient was anuric and clearly close to death. Initially she was placed on a conventional heart lung machine. An implantable ventricle pump was then tried, with modifications to the way it was implanted. It was placed into an aortic homograph attached as a third pulmonary vein to the left atrium, and was sited within the right pleural cavity. Such a device will support the circulation for 2–3 weeks. Systemic heparinization was not required. Initially there was no output at all from the patient's own left ventricle, but by 48 hours her heart was starting to pump and by the third day there was cardiac output. By the sixth day LV function was recovered and the device was removed. Two years later this patient has an essentially normal heart.

Another patient with end-stage dilated cardiomyopathy was treated with another device. This was an 8-year-old boy who needed a transplant but for whom a donor was not immediately available. An external right and left ventricular support device was used. The device was simple and rather crude but effective, and sustained the child's heart until a donor was found. A year after transplant he is back at school and very well.

New devices

The new generation pumps, which substitute for the left ventricle, are small, silent, require no anticoagulation and do not thrombose or cause haemolysis. The new Jarvik 2000 is an axial flow and propeller pump the size of an adult thumb. It spins at between 8000 and 14000 revolutions per minute and accelerates blood through a very narrow channel so fast that red cells are undamaged. It is implanted into the apex of the failing heart and offloads the heart to the descending thoracic aorta. Initial studies in sheep[7-9] revealed that, after 5 months, there is no thrombus in the pump. It is completely silent, and can only be heard with a stethoscope. Following the successful sheep studies, the Jarvik 2000 has also been implanted in human patients.[10] The size of the Jarvik 2000 pump is only the size of the inflow cannula of the Jarvik 7 pump and is the best available at the moment.

Problems

Infections via the power supply have been a constant worry with implanted cardiac assist devices. Transcutaneous power induction is not yet reliable and may not be so for some time. In cochlea implants, a carbon button is used to transmit power. Because it does not move in relation to the skin and because the scalp is highly vascular, there is virtual freedom from infection. A similar carbon pedestal has been designed for the heart Jarvik 2000.[8] The power comes up the neck into the carbon button and then to the external battery. In the sheep model there was 100% freedom from infection.[8] The transmitter resembles a hearing aid, and the power system is about the size of a portable telephone and can be worn on a belt. Even smaller versions have been developed for paediatric use.

The non-pulsatile devices mean that patients have to be managed without a pulse in the circulation. Lack of pulsatility does not seem to matter at all. Circulation filling pressures can be regulated via mixed venous oxygen saturation and urine output. Pulsatility does return when the device is removed. Sheep studies showed that, after 3 months chronic non-pulsatile flow, baroreceptor responses disappear but apparently return again after several hours following return to pulsatile flow.[7-9]

The future

Options for artificial hearts in the future probably will include permanent implants, bridges to transplantation and, perhaps more importantly, bridges to myocardial recovery. Such progress will largely depend upon molecular biology, an area that is evolving rapidly. Gene therapy to 'switch off' apoptosis may be one useful strategy. The process of apoptosis or programmed cell death, is responsible for the ventricular remodelling seen in heart failure. Inhibitors of apoptosis may help to sustain recovery when devices are removed. The concept of bridge to recovery may be particularly useful in patients with viral myocarditis. Patients with ischaemic cardiomyopathy can be supported following coronary bypass and virtually no patients need die from acute myocardial infarction. In the long term, idiopathic dilated cardiomyopathy, pericardial cardiomyopathy and cytotoxic drug-induced cardiomyopathy may also be amenable to support with these new devices (Box 3.2).

Box 3.2 Bridge to myocardial recovery

- Viral myocarditis
- Post cardiotomy support
- Acute cardiomyopathy
- Acute myocardial infarction

In the future a much wider application of blood pumps is likely to be seen. Devices will be implanted much earlier, before multisystems failure develops. They will soon be fully implantable, including the power source. Forty years ago pacemakers were huge but, in the same way as we have miniature pacemakers now for premature babies, we have miniature blood pumps, which are likely to completely transform the approach to heart failure in the next ten years.

Summary

Transplantation for end-stage heart failure is not always an option (Box 3.3). It is restricted by the availability of suitable donors, and there are problems associated with systemic infection, immunosuppression and rejection. Heart transplantation is irreversible. LVAD are readily available and often do not need anticoagulation. Progress has been made towards overcoming drive line infections and there is no rejection. The real benefit is recovery of the heart when it is rested with the LVAD.

Box 3.3 Heart transplant versus LVAD

Transplant

- Restricted to some patients
- Limitation of donors
- Immunosuppression
- Systemic infection
- Rejection
- Irreversible

LVAD

- Readily available
- Anticoagulation
- Drive line infection
- Recovery

References

1 Westaby S. Non-transplant surgery for heart failure. *Heart* 2000;**83**:603–10.
2 Westaby S. The need for artificial hearts. *Heart* 1996;**76**:200–6.
3 Morales DL, Argenziano M, Oz MC. Outpatients left ventricular assist devices support: a safe and economical therapeutic option for heart failure. *Prog Cardiovasc Dis* 2000;**43**:55–66.
4 McCarthy PM, Hoecher K. Clinically available intracorporeal left ventricular assist devices. *Prog Cardiovasc Dis* 2000;**43**:37–46.
5 Loisance DY, Jansen PG, Wheeldon DR, Portner PM. Long-term mechanical circulatory support with the wearable Novacor left ventricular assist system. *Eur J Cardiothorac Surg* 2000;**18**:220–4.
6 Noirhomme P, Jacquet L, Underwood M, El Khoury G, Goenen M, Dion R. The effect of chronic mechanical circulatory support of neuroendocrine activation in patients with end stage heart failure. *Eur J Cardiothorac Surg* 1999;**16**:63–7.
7 Westaby S, Katsumata T, Evans R, Pigott D, Taggart DP, Jarvik RK. The Jarvik 2000 Oxford system: increasing the scope of mechanical circulatory support. *J Thorac Cardiovasc Surg* 1997;**114**:467–74.
8 Jarvik RK, Westaby S, Katsumata T, Pigott D, Evans RD. LVAD power delivery: a percutaneous approach to avoid infection. *Ann Thorac Surg* 1998;**65**:470–3.
9 Westaby S, Katsumata T, Houel R, *et al.* Jarvik 2000 heart: potential for bridge to myocyte recovery. *Circulation* 1998;**98**:1568–74.
10 Westaby S, Banning AP, Jarvik RK *et al.* First permanent implant of the Jarvik 2000. *Lancet* 2000;**356**:900–3.

4: How to use echocardiography

ANDREW J BISHOP

Introduction

The aim of this article is to persuade you that an echocardiogram in the intensive care unit (ICU) can be useful and revealing. It will concentrate on the use of echo to identify causes of haemodynamic compromise and briefly discuss technological advances that may be relevant.

Haemodynamic compromise secondary to heart disease

Commonly, echocardiography in critically ill patients will reveal that the heart is enlarged. The heart may enlarge either to compensate for lack of contractile function or to accommodate the increased stroke volume from mitral or aortic valve regurgitation. However, in patients with primary ventricular disease it is also common to find a degree of functional or secondary mitral and aortic valve regurgitation. It is important to distinguish this from primary valvular heart disease. This distinction is difficult to make on clinical grounds since the physical signs can be very misleading. The crucial distinction is made on whether the systolic function of the ventricle is preserved or impaired. Many functional indices are quoted but these can be misleading and difficult to interpret (Box 4.1).

Box 4.1 Indices of left ventricular function

- Ejection fraction
- Fractional shortening
- Wall motion scoring
- E to A ratio

Indices of ventricular function

Systolic function is often quantified using the ejection fraction. Derivation of ejection fraction requires an accurate measurement of end-systolic and end-diastolic volumes, and technically this is not possible with conventional echo. For this reason an ejection fraction is more of an estimate than a measurement. In addition, the ejection fraction is sensitive to prevailing loading conditions. For this reason the ejection fraction should be treated as a rough guide rather than an exact index to be serially monitored. Other indices of ventricular systolic function are sometimes quoted and include fractional shortening and wall motion scoring. Fractional shortening is simply the ratio of end-systolic and end-diastolic dimensions at the base of the heart. This is insensitive to abnormalities of function that may occur at other areas towards the apex and is again only a rough estimate. Wall motion scoring assigns a score to each area of the LV myocardium according to whether it moves paradoxically, normally, or with reduced motion. Alternatively, it may be akinetic. The total motion score of the ventricle is the sum of the regional activities and, although it can be useful in the specialized circumstances of stress echocardiography, it does not contribute substantially to an understanding of resting systolic function.

Ventricular disease also often leads to abnormalities of ventricular filling, so-called diastolic dysfunction. The normal ventricle fills predominantly in a passive manner in the early phase, and, to a lesser extent actively, after atrial contraction. Recordings of flow across the mitral valve during diastole usually show a dominant early E-wave and a smaller A-wave. In most mild forms of ventricle disease the relaxation of the ventricle is impaired, and this interferes with the early filling of the ventricle. The balance is therefore shifted to the A-wave, which becomes dominant. However, as diastolic disease becomes more pronounced, the pressure in the ventricle during diastole increases, impeding filling owing to atrial contraction, and this pattern normalizes. As a rule of thumb, the presence of a significant or even dominant A-wave in the transmitral flow suggests that the LV end diastolic pressure is not markedly raised, and effectively excludes diastolic disease as a cause of significant haemodynamic compromise in intensive care.

Cardiac dimensions

In contrast to the indices described above, simple measurements of cardiac dimensions are of great value. A large heart has an increased end-diastolic dimension. If this increase is due to contractile failure, the end-systolic dimension is also increased. (This results, of course, in a reduction in the ejection fraction and the fractional shortening). However, if the heart is

23

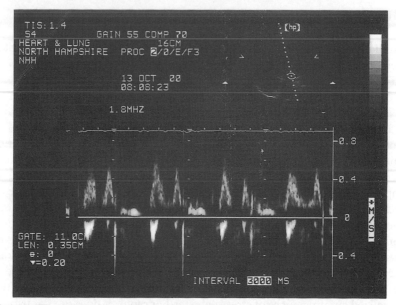

Figure 4.1 The normal pattern of E and A-wave filling of transmitral flow.

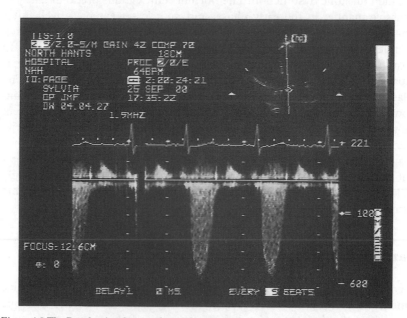

Figure 4.2 The Doppler signal across the aortic valve showing high velocity implying aortic stenosis.

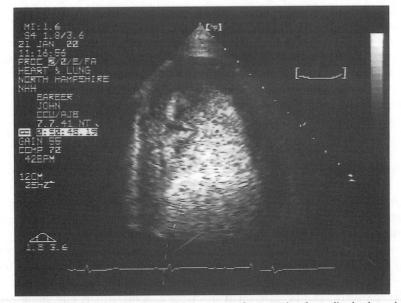

Figure 4.3 Left ventricular cavity filled with echo contrast demonstrating the cardiac border and the cavity.

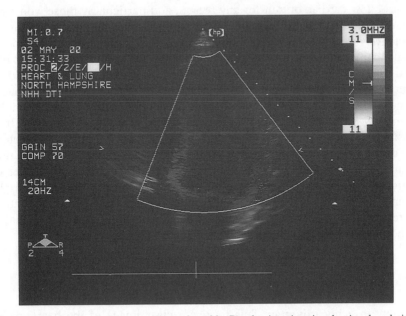

Figure 4.4 The left ventricular myocardium coloured by Doppler tissue imaging showing the velocity and direction.

25

enlarged because of valvular regurgitation, despite an increased end-diastolic dimension, the end-systolic dimension is reduced (reflecting the increased stroke volume). Thus, from an assessment of the end-systolic dimension, a distinction can be drawn between a heart with primary ventricular disease and a heart in which mitral or aortic valve regurgitation is the predominant problem. The latter group often require cardiac surgery. The former group fare poorly at cardiac surgery and should usually be protected from valve replacement.

Small hearts

Primary heart disease may be a cause of haemodynamic compromise in hearts that are not enlarged. This may be due to stenosis of the aortic or mitral valves, restrictive cardiomyopathy, pulmonary hypertension, or constrictive pericarditis. The use of Doppler echocardiography to measure the direction and velocity of flow across all four heart valves makes this diagnosis. A pressure gradient across the aortic, mitral, pulmonary, or tricuspid valve can be calculated from the Doppler trace, and significant pressure gradients usually imply haemodynamically important valvular stenosis. It is important to remember that when the cardiac output is low, pressure gradients may be correspondingly reduced. In patients therefore with a low cardiac output for any reason, and particularly those who have co-existent ventricular disease, valve stenosis may be severe, despite a relatively low gradient. This confusion can sometimes be reduced by calculating actual valve orifice areas, which are independent of cardiac output. However, the error in such calculations is high and they should be interpreted with some caution. The diagnoses of restrictive cardiomyopathy and constrictive pericarditis can be made reliably from abnormalities in the patterns of flow in diastole across the tricuspid and mitral valves. It is usually possible in addition to derive an estimate of pulmonary artery pressure from an echocardiogram, since minor tricuspid valve regurgitation can be detected in the majority of patients. The velocity of the jet of tricuspid regurgitation can be used to estimate the pressure in the right ventricle, since it is the difference between this pressure and the left atrial pressure that is driving the regurgitation. This technique is well validated and in common clinical use.

New technology

Often an echocardiogram fails to give a clear image of the heart in the intensive care unit. The image may be considerably improved by using the transoesophageal approach. Since the transoesophageal probe is posterior to the heart, it is particularly useful in assessing the anatomy of the aorta, the atria, and the aortic and mitral valves. The right side of the heart, the tricuspid and pulmonary valves, and left ventricle are less well imaged. Transoesophageal echo is particularly useful in the diagnosis of aortic and mitral valve disease, aortic dissection, and endocarditis. It has significant limitations in the assessment of LV function.

Intravenous contrast agents are now available that cross the pulmonary circulation and appear in all four chambers of the heart giving clear border recognition of endocardium. These agents are microbubbles of inert gas in a protein shell; they are harmless and transient. Use of these agents enormously improves picture quality in transthoracic echo; picture quality is often a major problem in the intensive care unit and contrast echo will prove a significant advance in this context.

New technology also allows derivation of Doppler signals, not only from the blood in the heart, but now also from the ventricular myocardium. These signals (Doppler tissue imaging) allow accurate regional quantification of velocity and direction of flow. They are likely to improve objective quantification of regional and global systolic function in the near future.

Conclusions

In normal cardiological practice, the echocardiogram is an indispensable tool in the diagnosis of haemodynamic disturbance. In the intensive care unit, where such disturbance is often much more critical, the echocardiogram can make crucial distinctions between the underlying causes of disease that require radically different approaches.

Further reading

1   Gmaurer G. Contrast echocardiography: clinical utility. *Echocardiography* 2000;**17**(6 part ii): S5–9.
2   Mulvagh SL. Myocardial perfusion by contrast echo. *Coronary Artery Dis* 2000;**11**:243–51.

5: Acute coronary syndromes

DAVID C CROSSMAN

Introduction

The acute coronary syndromes encompass Q wave or transmural (full thickness) myocardial infarction and the non-Q wave myocardial infarct/unstable angina interface. The pathogenesis of these syndromes is believed to involve disruption of an atherosclerotic plaque in the majority of cases. Coronary plaque disruption appears to be either plaque fissure or superficial plaque erosion resulting in thrombus accumulation in the artery and hence the acute coronary syndrome. This article will describe the therapeutic strategies available for this syndrome, which involves, in the main part, removal of the thrombus, prevention of further thrombus formation, and re-establishing adequate coronary blood flow.

Acute coronary syndromes

The acute coronary syndromes encompass three conditions: acute myocardial infarction, and the combination of non-Q wave myocardial infarction and unstable angina. These have some alternative names that are important to realize when you come to read the literature. Cardiologists tend to call acute myocardial infarction with ST elevation, transmural myocardial infarction. In contrast, non-Q wave infarction is referred to as sub-endocardial infarction. You may also find these described as ST elevation myocardial infarction (STEMI) or non-ST elevation myocardial infarction (non-STEMI) respectively. These are detailed in Box 5.1.

These conditions are, for the majority of patients, due to either rupture or erosion of atherosclerotic plaques within the coronary artery walls. Rupture or erosion of a plaque results in exposure of the contents of the plaque to the circulating blood resulting in clot formation and, when this happens in a coronary vessel, a coronary thrombus forms. Where a thrombus accumulates, of course, platelets also adhere to the subendothelial cell matrix. In addition, vasoconstriction either in the epicardial coronary segment, or downstream as a result of small changes in resistance vessels, contributes further to myocardial ischaemia. Cytokines, thromboxanes, 5-HT, and tissue factor also play a part.

Box 5.1 Acute coronary syndromes

- Acute myocardial infarction
  - Transmural myocardial infarction
  - Q wave myocardial infarction
  - ST elevation myocardial infarction (STEMI)
- Non-Q wave myocardial infarction
  - Sub-endothelial infarction
  - Non-ST elevation myocardial infarction (Non-STEMI)
- Unstable angina

Remember also that there are some rarer causes of coronary syndrome in patients with Q wave infarction, which do not result from plaque rupture or erosion, namely coronary emboli or coronary spasm. In patients with unstable angina there may be near zero coronary flow reserve because of the severity of their stable coronary plaque. It is very difficult to distinguish these causes clinically.

Therapeutic strategies in acute coronary syndromes

Given that, in the majority of patients, the cessation of coronary flow results from thrombus formation following atherosclerotic plaque rupture/erosion, the main therapeutic thrust is thrombus removal, inhibition of thrombus re-accumulation, and the restoration of blood flow. Agents along these lines include fibrinolytic drugs, antiplatelet agents, antithrombins, anti-ischaemics, and cardiac support (Box 5.2).

Box 5.2 Therapeutic strategies in coronary syndromes

- Antiplatelet agents
- Antithrombin agents
- Fibrinolytic agents
- Anti-ischaemic agents
- Cardiac support

It is worth re-emphasizing that acute or Q wave myocardial infarction differs very dramatically from non-Q wave infarction. There is a very high mortality risk in patients with acute myocardial infarct and the death rate from myocardial infarction remains between 18% and 20% in all comers. That contrasts with non-Q wave infarction, or unstable angina, patients who are not at immediate risk of death, although what the condition is presaging, of course, should be considered, since these patients may proceed to a cardiac event.

In the case of Q wave infarction, immediate revascularization, usually with aspirin adminstration and fibrinolytic therapy, is the established first-line treatment. Revascularization with percutaneous coronary intervention (PCI) confers a small advantage, perhaps owing to more complete vascularization as well as a reduction in the number of strokes that inevitably follow fibrinolytic therapy. PCI is not widely available for most acute myocardial infarction patients, and therefore new pharmaceutical agents for these Q wave infarcts are being tried. There have been a number of important clinical trials that have studied some of the available therapeutic agents.

In non-Q wave infarction/unstable angina, fibrinolytic therapy is proven to be of no use. Antiplatelet agents, however, do confer some benefit, and aspirin has been widely used in this condition. The development of more powerful antiplatelet agents, such as the glycoprotein IIb/IIIa antagonists and ADP-blockers have been studied. When such syndromes are treated, for clinical reasons, by percutaneous coronary revascularization techniques, IIb/IIIa antagonists undoubtedly reduce the complication rate and are of proven benefit. Trials of intravenous IIb/IIIa antagonist agents in non-Q wave infarction/unstable angina may reduce ischaemia and other early events, but observed benefits last only until day 30 after infarct. Nonetheless, these are now recommended in patients who are at high risk of developing complications. The use of an oral version of these agents, however, has been less convincing, and may even suggest more adverse events, perhaps owing to the pharmokinetics of the drugs.

Platelet glycoprotein IIb/IIIa is the receptor for fibrinogen. It is an integrin, a heterodimeric molecule comprising an α and a β chain. Because this is the fibrinogen receptor it forms the final pathway of platelet activation, adhesion, and aggregation. Glycoprotein IIb/IIIa inhibitors fall into three groups. The first group is the antibody agents such as Abciximab, an antibody against the IIIa sub-unit and which has non-specific effects outside the platelet IIb/IIIa receptor. It causes irreversible inhibition of platelet aggregation and is very expensive. There are also peptomimetics, which block the RGD binding site, of which Eptifibatide, also known as Integrilin, is the prototype. Non peptide agents include Lamifiban and Tirofiban.

The trials

There have been a number of trials of antiplatelet agents, which have been assessed in a meta-analysis.[1] The most important trials are known as the four Ps: Prism, Prism Plus, Paragon, and Pursuit, which were all reported in 1998. They have provided evidence of clear benefit. The largest of these studies, the Pursuit trial, investigated Integrilin and showed a statistically significant difference in death, myocardial infarction, and revascularization.[2] The Prism trial studied Tirofiban versus heparin and significance differences in the composite endpoints up to 48 hours were found.[3] In the Prism Plus study, Tirofiban plus heparin versus heparin alone showed some longer lasting beneficial differences in the composite endpoint.[4] Paragon was less convincing, but at lower doses of Lamifiban a beneficial effect in the composite endpoint for as long as six months was seen compared to patients treated with placebo.[5] The results of subset analysis is also of interest. The non-Q wave infarction/unsafe angina patients represent a non-homogeneous group of patients, ranging from people critically at risk to people who possibly have very little wrong with their heart. It is possible to distinguish between these types of patients using the cardiac specific marker, troponin. In the Prism trial of Tirofiban plus heparin versus heparin alone, troponin-positive patients, who received Tirofiban plus heparin, did better with this therapy than those who were troponin-positive and were treated with heparin alone.[6]

The use of low molecular weight heparins has been examined in unstable angina and non-STEMI. On the basis of two trials,[7, 8] there is a general consensus that the low molecular weigh heparin, Enoxaparin, has advantages over conventional unfractionated heparin. There are no trials comparing low molecular weight heparins and glycoprotein IIb/IIIa inhibitors.

Conclusion

The emerging areas for treatment in the next 5–10 years will be led primarily by changes in our improved understanding of acute coronary syndromes. Elucidation of events within the coronary vessel will almost certainly result in specific anti-inflammatory therapies for the vessel wall. Ongoing clinical trials of antibiotics in patients with unstable angina, following the suggestion that an infective agent may contribute to this condition, may also be fruitful.

References

1 Topol EJ, Byzova TV, Plow EF. Platelet GPIIb-IIIa blockers. *Lancet* 1999; **353**:227–31.
2 The PURSUIT Trial Investigators. Inhibition of platelet glycoprotein IIb/IIIa with eptifibatide in patients with acute coronary syndromes. Platelet glycoprotein IIb/IIIa in unstable angina: Receptor suppression using integrilin therapy. *NEJM* 1998;**339**:436–43.
3 Platelet Receptor Inhibition in Ischemic Syndrome Management (PRISM) Study Investigators. A comparison of aspirin plus tirofiban with aspirin plus heparin for unstable angina. *NEJM* 1998;**338**:1498–505.
4 Platelet Receptor Inhibition in Ischemic Syndrome Management in Patients Limited by Unstable Signs and Symptoms (PRISM-PLUS) Study Investigators. Inhibition of the platelet glycoprotein IIb/IIIa receptor with tirofiban in unstable angina and non-Q-wave myocardial infarction. *NEJM* 1998;**338**:1488–97.
5 Platelet IIb/IIIa Antagonism for the Reduction of Acute Coronary Syndrome Events in a Global Organization Network: The PARAGON Investigators. International, randomized, controlled trial of lamifiban (a platelet glycoprotein IIb/IIIa inhibitor), heparin, or both in unstable angina. *Circulation* 1998;**97**:2386–95.
6 Heeschen C, Hamm CW, Goldmann B, Deu A, Langenbrink L, White H: PRISM Study Investigators. Platelet Receptor Inhibition in Ischemic Syndrome Management D. Troponin concentrations for stratification of patients with acute coronary syndromes in relation to therapeutic efficacy of tirofiban. *Lancet* 1999;**354**:1757–62.
7 Antman EM, Cohen M, Radley D, *et al.* Assessment of the treatment effect of enoxaparin for unstable angina/non-Q-wave myocardial infarction. TIMI 11B-ESSENCE meta-analysis. *Circulation* 1999;**100**:1602–8.
8 Cohen M, Demers C, Gurfinkel EP, *et al.* A comparison of low-molecular-weight heparin with unfractionated heparin for unstable coronary artery disease. Efficacy and safety of subcutaneous enoxaparin in non-q-wave coronary events study group. *NEJM* 1997;**337**:447–52.

6: Managing arrhythmias

HUGH MONTGOMERY

Introduction

Cardiac dysrrhythmia is common in the critically ill and is associated with impaired prognosis. The diagnosis of the abnormal rhythm and its management can often be difficult. This article will provide a clear, concise hands-on approach to the management of various types of arrhythmia in patients on the intensive care unit (ICU).

Arrhythmia on ICU

Arrythmias are common, certainly dangerous, can be frightening, and are often poorly understood by most staff. Arrythmias occur frequently particularly as a result of the metabolic disturbances common to critical illness (Box 6.1). Most patients will be electrolytically deranged, with some degree of acid base disturbance. Microvascular or macrovascular ischaemic events cause damage to the heart, and there are generally increased circulating catecholamine levels (whether endogenous in response to fear or pain, or due to pharmacological administration). Together, these factors lead to the heart becoming more 'irritable'. It is therefore not surprising that arrhythmic problems occur so frequently. The question really is what to do about them.

Box 6.1 Mechanisms of arrhythmias on ICU

- Electrolyte disturbance
- Acid base disturbance
- Injury
- Cardiac irritability
  - Catecholamines/sedation
  - Hypoxaemia
  - Ischaemia

Simple rules for managing arrhythmias

There are a series of simple rules that can be used in the first-line management of arrhythmias on ICU. The first of these rules is that not all arrhythmias need to be treated at all. If your patient is haemodynamically compromised, with poor cardiac output and blood pressure, and all the complications that go with it, then it is clear that prompt action is required. If a patient is likely to become compromised, is in atrial fibrillation, perhaps aged 70 or over, with poor ventricular function, and borderline blood pressure, then some form of action is likely to be required soon. However, if your patient is not haemodynamically compromised, and unlikely to become so, antidysrrhythmic treatment is not needed at all. It is worth pointing out that every antidysrrhythmic agent is pro-arrhythmic at the right dose and in the right patient. It can be a difficult decision deciding not to treat, but this may in fact be sensible.

Rule two is that electricity is safe and drugs are dangerous. There is not an antidysrrhythmic drug known that does not also have potential to cause dysrrhythmia. Electricity, safely and appropriately applied is a very safe form of therapy, whether it be DC cardioversion or pacing. If you treat your patients with one drug that does not work, you have got a problem because, as soon as you try another drug, it is impossible to know whether the continued dysrrhythmia is now actually due to the combination of drugs rather than the primary problem. If you have a choice always choose electricity over drugs.

Rule three says that if your patient has a tachycardia, whatever the cause, and is compromised, administer a shock. Digoxin is the exception to the 'avoid drugs' rule. It is a much forgotten agent, very safe, and has a wide therapeutic index. It is the only antidysrrhythmic that is actually a positive inotrope, rather than a negative inotrope. Adenosine is also useful, because of its rapid onset of action and very rapid degradation.

Rule four is that if you have got time, you should try to correct any metabolic abnormalities. Lack of attention to metabolic disruption creates a lower threshold for dysrrhythmia, and failing to attend to these metabolic abnormalities may result in dysrrhythmias that do not respond. If you are short of time, treat the dysrrhythmia and the metabolic compromise at the same time.

It is safe to assume that most critically ill patients are magnesium deficient at the cellular level. Rule five is that giving magnesium to almost every patient who is pro-arrhythmic, at a rate of 20 mM over 15 minutes or so, and keeping plasma potassium levels at between 4·8–5·5 mmol/litre, is a good strategy.

All ischaemic patients should have their ischaemia treated, prior to correction of the dysrrhythmia if possible, or simultaneously in the presence of haemodynamic compromise. Although not classically anti-arrhythmic, nitrates and β-blockers may thus be antiarrhythmic through reductions in ischaemic burden. Balloon pumps are also excellent when you are faced with ischaemia and no other means of improving coronary blood flow.

The last rule, which should probably be the first rule, is that central lines can cause arrhythmias. It is simple enough to draw back the central line a few centimetres or remove the pulmonary artery catheter, and these simple measures often resolve the problem.

Specific dysrrhythmias

Atrial fibrillation

The same rules can be applied to patients in atrial fibrillation (AF): if the rate is fast and the patient is haemodynamically compromised, the approach should be to administer a DC shock. Remember to ensure adequate sedation, since DC shock is unpleasant when the patient is fully conscious. Conventional paddle position is less than ideal for cardioverting atrial fibrillation at lower energies to critically ill patients, especially when their lungs may be highly inflated. The choice of a posterior paddle position is helpful. It has been suggested that there is a risk with digoxin in these patients. Such risks are only worth considering if digoxin levels are very high, in toxic ranges, and potassium levels are very low. If DC cardioversion is not possible, rapid rate control might be also be appropriate, with digoxin, amiodarone or a β-blocker.

If the patient is compromised and shocking fails, and this is not uncommon, metabolic abnormalities and inadequate filling need to be corrected. Once you have done these two things, try again with DC shocking. In the event of continued failure, give 300–400 mg amioderone over 5 to 10 minutes with constant monitoring, then shock again.

If your patient is in AF but is not haemodynamically compromised then take time to think about what to do. If this is a new acute AF, then clearly it is to the patient's benefit in the longer term to be in sinus rhythm during the stay on the ICU. The best approach in this situation is to correct any metabolic abnormalities, increasing particularly potassium and magnesium, correct any filling deficits, adjust line position, and perhaps the problem will resolve itself. If this is not the case and the patient is ventilated and heavily sedated, it is likely that sinus rhythm can be restored simply with a DC shock. Of course, the same can be achieved with a number of other agents and in expert hands on a coronary unit, there are several options. In patients on a general ICU, however, coronary status and ventricular function may be unknown, in which case you are limited to shocking or giving amioderone.

Trials of magnesium in intensive care unit patients have shown that AF can be largely treated just by using magnesium – certainly in the postoperative patient. The causes of magnesium deficit are shown in Box 6.2 to demonstrate how incredibly common magnesium deficiency can be, explaining why just giving magnesium to critically ill patients with dysrrhythmia is often all that is required.

Box 6.2 Causes of magnesium deficiency

- Diarrhoea
- Diuretics
- Diet
- Diabetes
- Alcohol
- Drugs

In the absence of haemodynamic compromise and suspicion of chronic AF, then rate control and, in the longer term, anticoagulation, is probably all that is needed. Of course, there is an acute thrombotic risk in the absence of anticoagulation, but this is generally small in the absence of mitral stenosis, severe hypertrophy, or poor ventricular function. Achieving good rate control may be all that is required, and digoxin is not a bad first-line choice since, as stated earlier, it is not a negative inotrope and its therapeutic window is relatively large unless a patient is in renal failure. To achieve reasonable rate control a fairly large dose at a fairly fast rate will be required, with monitoring.

Supraventricular tachycardia

As before, if patients are haemodynamically compromised, the first approach is DC shock, attending to the metabolic derangement, correct filling, adjusting the line position and moving on to adenosine therapy and further shocking if this fails. Adenosine is, however, very rapidly acting and can be given if it is immediately available. If haemodynamic compromise is present, regardless of whether this is ventricular tachycardia (VT) or supraventricular tachycardia (SVT), then DC shock is the first approach.

Ventricular tachycardia

Most cases of broad complex tachycardia are VT, particularly in the presence of ischaemia. Confirmation requires the presence of independent

P-wave activity, or capture or fusion beats on a rhythm strip. In compromised patients in VT, drugs alone work in only 40% of patients as a first-line treatment, especially in the absence of correction of all the factors that might be leading to the ventricular tachycardia in the first place. Obviously, once sinus rhythm is restored with DC shock, this is a different matter. Once out of VT, sinus rhythm can be held with an intravenous infusion of lignocaine or amiodarone or, if ventricular function is adequate enough, β-blockers. As a final resort, pace termination can be attempted using a pacemaker box set at a rate about 10% slower than the rate of the patient's intrinsic rhythm, to capture the ventricle. When the ventricle is 'captured', the rate on the monitor will drop to that at which you are pacing, and the QRS morphology is likely to change. There are then two choices: you can either decrease the rate very slowly or switch the pacemaker off completely. In the majority of cases, the dysrrhythmia will be extinguished.

It is also possible to achieve the same by setting the pacemaker rate faster than the patient's rate. There are advantages to this: one is that it is easier to break into the cardiac cycle. However, this is not recommended, since there are risks of acceleration of the rhythm, and the general ICU is not the place to do it. More sophisticated pacemaker boxes that allow the planting of an extra beat at different stages of the dysrrhythmia are generally not available.

Bradycardia

There are a number of causes of bradycardia. These include electrolyte abnormalities and poisoning with drugs such as digoxin. If patients are compromised and bradycardia is a continuing problem, then pace the patient. It is probably important to remember when using pacing that two chambers are indeed better than one, especially in the elderly and in people with slightly thicker ventricles or diastolic stiffness. These patients are often much better having AV synchrony. Remember too that chronic bradycardia may cause trouble when you are pacing, since the patient's escape rhythm may be extinguished, resulting in pacemaker dependence.

Other

There are one or two other indications for pacing. If you have a febrile patient with an increasing PR interval, the diagnosis until determined otherwise is endocarditis with an aortic root abscess. You might ask why you should pace someone with a lengthening PR interval. Quite simply these are the patients who, when they develop complete heart block, go into ventricular asystole. For these reasons, it is much better in such patients to pace earlier.

The other situation where prophylactic pacing may be indicated is trifascicular block (long PR interval, with right bundle-branch block and left axis deviation, or long PR with left bundle-branch block). Here, one is only running on a single fascicle. If the patient would be at risk if complete heart block were to develop (e.g. very poor ventricle), then a temporary pacing wire might be considered.

Conclusion

This article has, I hope, provided a practical approach to the understanding of dysrrhythmias, and to their management. The message is to remember electrolytes, oxygenation, magnesium, potassium, line position, ischaemia, sedation, and analgesia – in all patients and at the same time.

Further reading

1 Ramsay JG. Cardiac management in the ICU. *Chest* 1999;**115**(Suppl.): 38S–144S.
2 Lee SH, Chang CM, Lu MJ, *et al*. Intravenous amiodarone for prevention of atrial fibrillation after coronary artery bypass grafting. *Ann Thorac Surg* 2000;**70**:157–61.
3 Johnson RG, Shafique T, Sirois C, Weintraub RM, Comunale ME. Potassium concentrations and ventricular ectopy: a prospective, observational study in post-cardiac surgery patients. *Crit Care Med* 1999;**27**:2430–4.
4 Creswell LL. Postoperative atrial arrhythmias: risk factors and associated adverse outcomes. *Semin Thorac Cardiovasc Surg* 1999;**11**:303–7.
5 Francis GS. Cardiac complications in the intensive care unit. *Clinics Chest Med* 1999;**20**:269–85.

7: Estimation of cardiac output

MAX M JONAS

Introduction

One of the major problems in assessing circulatory disturbances in a patient is that blood pressure is frequently used as a substitute for flow. Unfortunately, as the two are not directly related, there is no correlation between flow and pressure. Furthermore it is incredibly difficult to *clinically* estimate cardiac output from clinical data alone.[1,2]

A plethora of methods have been developed to estimate cardiac output. Each method has potential for measurement errors and a requirement for technical expertise that may limit its utility. Another major consideration is the degree of invasiveness required to obtain a cardiac output determination and the incremental risk to the patient.

This article will describe methods currently available for the estimation of cardiac output and will concentrate particularly on lithium dilution and a novel pulse waveform analysis technique as a safer alternative to thermodilution.

Cardiac output and blood pressure

Despite a multitude of techniques for estimating cardiac output, its determination is not a direct measurement but only an estimate. In physiological terms a measurement is a directly obtained value (i.e. pressure from a transducer) and an estimate is an indirect value derived from a number of measurements.

Clinically, measurements of blood pressure are easy to obtain, whilst estimation of cardiac output is indirect and more difficult. This means that clinicians rely heavily on measurement of pressure as an index to perfusion, although available data actually show that there is virtually no correlation between observed changes in pressure and changes in flow.

Physiologically and theoretically, perfusion – or blood flow – is the variable that doctors who are looking after critically ill patients should attempt to manipulate. The caveat here is that knowledge of flow in isolation of the haemoglobin concentration and arterial saturation may be misleading. Cellular viability depends on oxygen delivery (cardiac output × arterial oxygen content) not just cardiac output. A recent unpublished study clearly demonstrates that despite apparently adequate cardiac output in intensive care patients, 23% had suboptimal oxygen delivery owing to anaemia and\or respiratory failure (Bruce R, Jonas M, O'Brien T, Band D, personal communication.).

So how can an estimation of cardiac output be generated? There are three main methods for determination of cardiac output and each of these is described briefly below. The ideal characteristics for estimation of cardiac output are given in Box 7.1.

Box 7.1 Ideal characteristics of a method to determine cardiac ouput

- Non-invasive
- Applicable to many patients
- Applicable over a wide range of flow
- Accurate (compared to other techniques)
- Reproducible
- Easy to use
- Rapid data acquisition
- Cost effective

Fick equation

A method of estimating cardiac output was described by Fick in 1870. Fick suggested that that cardiac output could be calculated from the arteriovenous oxygen content difference and oxygen consumption. This requires measurement of oxygen consumption by spirometry and oxygen content by blood gas analysis. The requirement for a mixed venous sample necessitates a pulmonary artery catheter. Although the estimation of cardiac output by the Fick equation is probably regarded as the 'gold standard', and can certainly be very accurate, it requires a great degree of technical skill and relies on other measurements, each with potential errors. It is clearly not feasible as a technique that can be used routinely. Several devices use variants of the Fick principle.

Doppler echocardiography

Ultrasonic Doppler velocimetry in conjunction with ultrasonic echo imaging of the descending aorta has been proposed as a valid non-invasive technique for measurement of descending aortic blood flow.[2,3] With experience, Doppler estimation of cardiac output is an accurate tool. However, insertion of the oesophageal probe requires an intubated patient, and certain anatomical and mathematical assumptions must be made to extrapolate the total flow from the descending aortic flow. The process is entirely user dependent, requiring practice and pattern recognition of the Doppler signal. Rotation of the probe in the oesophagus changes the estimate of descending aortic flow and limits the concept of continuous cardiac output monitoring.

Indicator dilution

Dye dilution

The bolus indicator dilution technique for measurement of cardiac output was originally described by Henriques and further developed by Hamilton *et al.*, based on the concept of the dilution of a known amount of indicator.[4] A dye such as indocyanine green is injected into a central catheter and arterial blood is sampled for measurement of dye content. Cardiac output can be estimated using the quantity of dye injected divided by the area under the arterial dilution curve.

Similar to the Fick method, this technique can be accurate but is technically difficult and time consuming. Thermodilution, in which cold or heat is used as the marker, is now the most commonly used method. Originally described by Fegler, this method was adapted for use in man by Bradley and Branthwaite in 1968 and further modified for commercial use by Swan and Ganz in 1971.

Thermodilution

The thermodilution technique is based on the indicator dilution method. Three different thermodilution techniques are in clinical use. All use a thermal indicator (cold or heat) injected into the right heart and sensed either in the pulmonary artery (Swan–Ganz pulmonary artery catheter) or in the aorta (transpulmonary thermodilution).

The pulmonary artery catheter is the most commonly used clinical device for estimating cardiac output. In this case, a known volume of cold dextrose is injected into the right atrium, and the temperature change in the pulmonary artery is sensed by a thermistor on the side of the catheter.

The cardiac output is calculated from the temperature time curve. Pulmonary arterial thermodilution has several disadvantages and its use is currently the subject of considerable scrutiny.[5-7]

Apart from technical limitations to cardiac output estimation, the greatest problem with the Swan–Ganz catheter is the catheter-related morbidity and mortality. This technique clearly can only be applied to patients on intensive care units. There is therefore an urgent need for the development of a simple, safe, robust, and inexpensive method for determination of cardiac output.

Lithium dilution cardiac output

Lithium is a good alternative marker for the indicator dilution method of estimating cardiac output for a number of reasons. It is safe, non-toxic in small doses, and easy to measure using an ion-selective electrode. There is no significant first pass loss from the circulation and it is rapidly redistributed. Furthermore, unless the patient is on lithium therapy for mania, it is not present in the body, and this produces an indicator with an extremely high signal to noise ratio. Lithium is a commonly used drug in the practice of psychiatry and its pharmacology and pharmacokinetic profiles are therefore well known.

Lithium chloride (adult dose 0.15 mmol) is injected as an intravenous bolus and its concentration time curve is measured in arterial plasma by withdrawing arterial blood at 4 ml/min past a lithium-selective electrode attached to the arterial line. The cardiac output is calculated from the lithium dose and the area under the concentration time curve prior to recirculation. The design of the ion-selective electrode and the model used to calculate cardiac output has been described in detail.[8-10]

A series of experiments in 40 patients, who had undergone cardiopulmonary bypass for cardiac surgery, showed good agreement between the thermodilution and lithium dilution methods for measuring cardiac output, and the data suggested greater precision with the lithium technique.[12] The lithium technique has also been used in children: 17 children were studied and lithium dilution measurements were compared with transpulmonary thermodilution. As discussed above, this technique is similar to thermodilution but the thermistor is placed in the aorta via the femoral artery rather than the pulmonary artery. Again agreement was very good between lithium and thermodilution.[11]

Larger animals have also been studied including horses, dogs, and a giraffe, to ensure that the technique remained valid, despite vast differences in body weight and shape – the weights studied ranged from about a 2 kg baby up to a 558 kg horse![12]

Obviously most critically ill patients have central venous access as well as arterial access, but there would be a considerable advantage to being able to use lithium dilution cardiac output via a peripheral vein in patients without central venous lines. A study of stable patients on the intensive care unit, with both central and peripheral lines showed that the correlation between peripherally and centrally injected lithium dilution was excellent, and it is clear that only a peripheral line and an arterial line is needed to estimate cardiac output using this technique.[13] As with all indicator dilution techniques, abnormal vascular shunts would result in errors of measurement and, additionally, this technique cannot be used in patients on chronic lithium therapy because of background lithium levels.

The future

If one of the significant triggers for organ failure is hypoperfusion then the goal of haemodynamic monitoring must be to ensure the adequacy of perfusion in patients who appear stable, and to detect *early* any inadequacies in others. This therefore leads to a requirement for a real time continuous estimate of cardiac output. The benefits and ideal characteristics of a real time system are shown in Boxes 7.2 and 7.3.

Box 7.2 Benefits of continuous cardiac output

- Early warning monitoring
- Rational fluid and drug administration
- Reduced work of healthcare staff
- Decreased procedural complications, e.g. bolus injections

Box 7.3 Ideal characteristics of a continuous cardiac output device

- Non-invasive
- Automatic and non-operator dependent
- Accurate (compared to other techniques)
- Continuous, real time data display
- Easy to use
- No calibration required
- Cost effective

Three systems are registered in the UK that attempt to estimate cardiac output on a continuous basis.

Vigilance™

The Vigilance™ (Edwards Lifesciences) uses a thermal approach with a modified pulmonary artery catheter. A heating coil in the right ventricle heats the blood in a pseudorandom sequence. The resulting temperature change is detected downstream in the pulmonary artery and the cross-correlation of the detected temperature change and the heating sequence generates a thermodilution curve.[14] This is probably the most widely used system clinically at present but the major drawback remains the necessity for pulmonary artery catheterization. The signal to noise ratio is poor with temperature changes measured in fractions of a degree, and the system is not truly continuous as it takes a variable time to update.

PICCO™

Two newer systems that avoid pulmonary artery catheterization have recently become available. The PICCO™ system (Pulsion Medical Systems) uses transpulmonary thermodilution to calibrate a pulse contour analysis algorithm of the arterial waveform. The morphology of the aortic waveform is analysed via a femoral artery catheter, and an attempt to delineate the ejection systolic area (i.e. pressure waveform between the start of ventricular ejection and the dichrotic notch) is made by a computer algorithm. Once the algorithm is calibrated, changes in the ejection systolic area and the heart rate are displayed as changes in cardiac output. Clinical experience of this system is developing but arrhythmias, unusual waveform morphology, and certain vasoactive drugs can produce errors in the estimation.[15] The interval between calibrations has yet to be determined but may have to be relatively frequent in unstable patients.

PulseCO

The PulseCO system (LiDCO Cardiac Sensors Ltd) is a new approach to continuous real time cardiac output. This system uses radial artery waveform analysis, derived from the patient monitor, and an algorithm that calculates the cardiac power using autocorrelation. This method is not waveform morphology – or area-dependent, but requires calibration with the lithium dilution method. The system is still under clinical scrutiny but early results from the Berlin Heart Institute and Southampton General Hospital are extremely encouraging especially in unstable patients. This PulseCO system has also approached the display and interpretation of continuous data in a novel way, potentially enabling staff with varying levels of expertise to interpret the data.

References

1   Tibby SM, Hatherill M, Marsh MJ, Murdoch IA. Clinicians' abilities to estimate cardiac index in ventilated children and infants. *Arch Dis Child* 1997;**77**:516–18.

2   Freund PR. Modifications in the transesophageal Doppler: comparison with thermodilution measurement of cardiac output in anesthetized man. *Anesthesiology* 1996;**65**:A144.

3   Singer M,Clarke J,Bennett ED. Continuous haemodynamic monitoring by oesophageal Doppler. *Crit Care Med* 1989;**17**:447–52.

4   Hamilton WF, Moore JW, Kinsman JM, Spurling RG. Studies on the circulation IV. Further analysis of the injection methods and of changes in hemodynamics under physiological and pathological conditions. *Am J Physiol* 1932;**99**:534–51.

5   Davies GG, Jebson PJR, Glasgow BM, *et al*. Continous Fick cardiac output compared to thermodilution cardiac output. *Crit Care Med* 1986;**14**:881

6   Connors AF Jr, Speroff T, Dawson NV, *et al*. The effectiveness of right heart catheterization in the initial care of critically ill patients. *J Am Med Assoc* 1996;**18**(276):889–97.

7   Dalen JE, Bone RC. Is it time to pull the pulmonary artery catheter? *J Am Med Assoc* 1996;**276**:916–18.

8   Linton RAF, Band DM, Haire KM. A new method of measuring cardiac output in man using lithium diliution. *Br J Anaesth* 1993;**71**:262–6.

9   Band DM, Linton RAF, Jonas MM, Linton NWF. The shape of indicator curves used for cardiac output measurement in man. *J Physiol* 1997;**498**:225–9.

10 Linton RAF, Band DM, O'Brien T, Jonas MM, Leach R. Lithium dilution cardiac output measurement: a comparison with thermodilution. *Crit Care Med* 1997;**25**:1796–800.

11 Linton RAF, Jonas MM, Tibby SM, *et al*. Cardiac output measured by lithium dilution and transpulmonary thermodilution in patients in a pediatric intensive care unit. *Intensive Care Med* 2000;**26**:1507–11.

12 Linton RAF, Young LE, Marlin DJ, *et al*. Cardiac output measured by lithium dilution, thermodilution and transesophageal Doppler echocardiography in anesthetized horses. *Am J Vet Res* 2000;**61**:731–7.

13 Jonas MM, Kelly FE, Linton RAF, Band DM, O'Brien TK, Linton NWF. A comparison of lithium dilution cardiac output measurements made using central and antecubital venous injection of lithium chloride. *J Clin Monit Comp* 1999;**15**:525–8.

14 Yelderman M, Ramsay M, Quinn M, Paulsen A, McKown R, Gillman P. Continuous thermodilution cardiac output measurements in intensive care patients. *J Cardiothorac Vasc Anaesth* 1992;**6**:270–4.

15 Rodig G, Prasser C, Keyl C, Liebold A, Hobbhahn J. Continuous cardiac output measurement: pulse contour analysis vs thermodilution technique in cardiac surgical patients. *Br J Anaesth* 1999;**82**:525–30.

8: The heart and vasculature in sepsis and septic shock (Gilston Lecture)

JOSEPH E PARRILLO

Introduction

Septic shock is the commonest cause of death on intensive care units. Although sepsis usually results in low systemic vascular resistance, there is strong evidence for depressed myocardial function. In this article the incidence and pathogenesis of septic shock and the characteristic cardiovascular abnormalities are described, in addition to current therapeutic approaches.

Incidence of sepsis and septic shock

The incidence of sepsis and septic shock has been increasing steadily over the past 60 years and all estimates suggest that this rise will continue. It is the most common cause of death in intensive care units in the USA and the numbers for Western Europe are similar.[1] The increase in incidence is probably due to a combination of reasons, including greater use of invasive devices, immunosuppressive and cytotoxic drugs, increased antibiotic resistance, and increasing age of the population.[2] Of the half a million people who develop sepsis every year, about half develop refractive hypotension – 'septic shock' – and between approximately 100 000 and 200 000 people die of this disease every year. The mortality rate of sepsis as a whole depends, of course, upon the severity of illness; however, when those patients with septic shock are considered, the death rate varies between 30% and 70%.

Septic shock is a unique form of shock and probably the least understood from a haemodynamic perspective. Cardiogenic, extracardiac obstructive and oligaemic shock all produce the acute phase of the syndrome of shock through decreased cardiac output. Septic shock, however, is a distributive form of shock, and results in markedly decreased systemic vascular resistance and a generalized disturbance of blood flow.

The classifications of different types of shock are given in Box 8.1. In most volume-loaded patients with septic shock, cardiac output is either normal or elevated, such that the hypotension results from reduced vascular resistance and not low cardiac output. In the 1950s it was usual practice not to fluid-resuscitate patients with sepsis and septic shock, and during that period the mortality rate was about 90%.

Box 8.1 Classification of forms of shock

- Cardiogenic shock
  - Myopathic shock (reduced systolic function)
    - acute myocardial function
    - dilated cardiomyopathy
    - myocardial depression in septic shock
  - Mechanical shock
    - mitral regurgitation
    - ventricular septal defect
    - ventricular aneurysm
  - Left ventricular outflow obstruction shock
    - aortic stenosis
    - hypotrophic cardiomyopathy
  - Arrhythmic shock
- Extracardiac obstructive shock
  - Pericardial tamponade
  - Constrictive pericarditis
  - Pulmonary embolism
  - Severe pulmonary hypertension
    - Coarctation of the aorta
- Oligaemic shock
  - Haemorrhage
  - Fluid depletion
- Distributive shock
  - Septic shock
  - Toxic products, e.g. overdose
  - Anaphylaxis
  - Neurogenic shock
- Endocrine shock

Pathogenesis of sepsis

The pathogenetic mechanisms of the cardiovascular disturbance in septic shock are complex. Figure 8.1 illustrates schematically the mechanisms that are thought to be involved. The process of sepsis begins with a focus of infection, such as an abscess, pneumonitis, peritonitis, cellulites, etc. The offending micro-organisms may invade the bloodstream, resulting in positive blood cultures and mediator release, or, alternatively, the organisms proliferating in the site of infection may directly lead to the release of various mediators into the bloodstream. This includes exotoxins, endotoxin, and other products from bacteria, or host-derived mediators, such as cytokines and components of the complement cascade. There are many mediator molecules released, which are involved in the pathogenesis of sepsis and which profoundly affect both the vascular system and the myocardium itself.

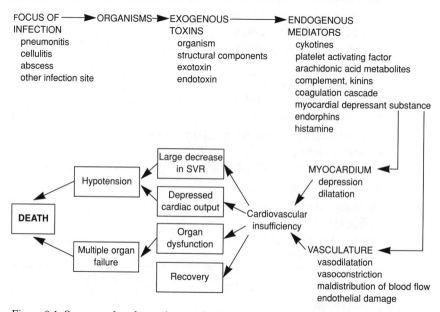

Figure 8.1 Sequence of pathogenetic steps leading from a focus of infection to cardiovascular dysfunction and shock during human sepsis. Data reproduced with permission from Parrillo JE. Ann Intern Med *1990;113:227–42.*[3]

Septic shock

The vascular and myocardial effects of systemically produced mediators lead to the development of generalized cardiovascular derangements and the syndrome of septic shock. For each 100 patients admitted to state-of-the-art intensive care facilities, in approximately 50, reversal of the shock as a result of aggressive early fluid resuscitation therapy means that these patients survive. The remaining 50 patients do not survive, as a result of refractory hypotension or progressive sequential loss of organ function, called multi-organ dysfunction syndrome or MODS. Unresponsive hypotension is primarily due to low systemic vascular resistance, typically not able to be corrected by any therapeutic intervention. In less than 10% of patients, the hypotension is due to low cardiac output, or uncompensated myocardial depression. MODS commonly affects the lungs, kidney, gut, liver, heart, and central nervous system, leading to organ failure and ultimately death. Low cardiac output is uncommon even in late stages of septic shock, and persistently elevated cardiac output has been shown to be associated with non-survival. This is demonstrated in the study by Parker *et al*[4] and illustrated in Figure 8.2. This study revealed that patients with septic shock who do not survive have persistence of the characteristic hyperdynamic haemodynamic profile, i.e. increased heart rate, high cardiac output and increased systemic vascular resistance, whilst in patients who survive, haemodynamics begin to return towards normal within 24 hours. Cut off values for these parameters could be used to predict survival and guide therapy.[4]

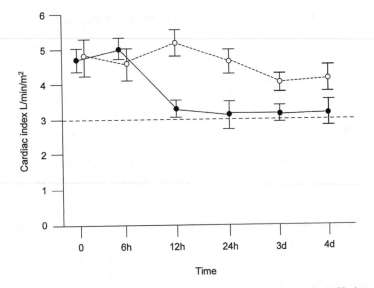

Figure 8.2 Serial mean cardiac index in survivors and non-survivors of septic shock. Horizontal line is the mean cardiac index in healthy people. The cardiac index returns to normal in survivors (closed circles) but remains increased in non-survivors (open circles). Data reproduced with permission from Parker MM, et al. Crit Care Med 1987;15:923–9.[4]

End diastolic volume index and left ventricular (LV) ejection fraction index provide a more accurate assessment of ventricular performance than blood pressure. During the acute phase of septic shock, the ejection fraction, associated with a dilated left ventricle, decreases to approximately 35% and the diastolic volume is increased. However, this low ejection fraction is transient in patients who recover, and the ejection fraction returns to normal. In survivors of septic shock, end diastolic volume index and ejection fraction show a negative correlation, which is lost in patients who do not survive.[5] Thus in non-survivors the decreased ejection fraction is not consistently associated with ventricular dilatation, and may lead to inadequate filling of the left ventricle, poor stroke volume, and therefore low cardiac output. This may contribute to death in these patients.

This scenario of decreased ventricular ejection fraction occurs essentially in every patient who develops sepsis and septic shock. Some patients will have low pulmonary artery occlusion pressure when a pulmonary artery (PA) catheter is inserted, but fluid resuscitation will lead to the development of a high cardiac output/low resistance haemodynamic profile. Some patients have such severe myocardial depression that cardiac output is actually low but, as stated previously, this is relatively uncommon, although it is does sometimes occur.

Mediators of myocardial depression in sepsis

Bacterial products

The question then arises as to whether these characteristic cardiovascular abnormalities are related to known immune or inflammatory mediators. Endotoxin is a lipopolysaccharide associated with the cell membranes of gram negative bacteria, and which elicits a shock-like state, with organ dysfunction and poor perfusion in animal models. In patients with septic shock and positive blood cultures, detectable circulating concentrations of endotoxin are correlated with increased lactate levels, lower systemic vascular resistance, and depressed ventricular ejection fraction. Indeed, mortality was also increased: 39% in patients with endotoxaemia compared to 7% in those without.[6] Since it is clear that endotoxin is important, the link between endotoxin and the cardiovascular abnormalities characteristic of sepsis and septic shock was studied further. Remember these cardiovascular abnormalities are high output, low resistance, decreased ejection fraction, and ventricular dilatation.

Small intravenous doses of purified endotoxin were therefore administered to human volunteers.[7] Such small doses can be safely administered, and subjects merely develop a transient flu-like illness, with mild fever. The study showed that endotoxin induces tachycardia, increases cardiac index and reduces blood pressure and systemic vascular index, without affecting stroke volume. Although these changes were not apparent clinically, they were easily detected using careful cardiovascular monitoring. The results of this study provided a clear link between endotoxin and myocardial depression, such that the haemodynamic profile similar to that seen in human sepsis, with a high cardiac index, low systemic vascular resistance, and a reversible depression of ventricular function, was produced by endotoxin. Endotoxin is therefore a major mediator of sepsis-induced cardiovascular dysfunction.

Animal models of sepsis have been used extensively to answer some of the questions related to myocardial depression. These models include intravenous administration of live bacteria or endotoxin itself, or, more physiologically, implantation of blood clots in the peritoneum, which then serve as the focus of infection shown in Figure 8.1. Using such models, it was determined that the myocardial depression was dose dependent, such that the higher the bacterial or endotoxin load, the more pronounced the myocardial depression. In addition, it was also shown that myocardial depression was similar, regardless of whether bacteria were gram positive or gram negative, and even dead bacteria caused similar abnormalities. These important studies indicated that, although endotoxin could lead to the cardiovascular derangements of septic shock, it is certainly not the only mediator. It is only one of many bacterially derived substances that contribute to the manifestations of sepsis and septic shock.[8]

Host-derived mediators

Studies using cultured myocytes have also been useful in answering some of the questions relating to myocardial depression in sepsis. Such rat myocytes in culture in the laboratory can either be allowed to beat spontaneously or can be paced. Video microscopy can be used to monitor myocardial cell performance, i.e. contraction independent of preload, after-load or heart rate, measured as shortening, and motion detection can be used to determine single cell ejection fraction accurately. It was shown that exposing these cells to serum from patients with acute septic shock induced cardiac myocyte contractile depression.[9] Serum from patients with septic shock depressed myocyte contractile function on average by about 40% and, following recovery, this depressant activity disappeared. It was also shown that the ejection fraction in septic shock patients, determined by radionuclide scan, correlated significantly with rat cardiac myocyte shortening *in vitro* in response to that patient's serum. Clearly this is very important to the clinician, since it demonstrated elegantly a strong link between *in vivo* cardiac function and a myocardial depressant substance circulating in patients' blood.

Another series of studies by Kumar *et al*[10] showed that the myocyte depressive effect of septic serum seen in rat cells *in vitro* could be mimicked in a dose-dependent fashion by tumour necrosis factor α (TNFα) and interleukin-1β (IL-1β), and the effect was synergistic. Many other cytokines, including interferonγ, IL-2, IL-4, IL-6, IL-8 and IL-10 were also tested, but failed to have the same myocardial depressant effect. The effect of TNFα and IL-1β occurred within 10 minutes, indicating that this could not be explained by *de novo* protein synthesis. Other studies, however, have also showed a delayed and prolonged depressant effect of TNFα and IL-1β on myocardium *in vitro*, beginning hours after exposure, persisting for several days and suggesting that synthesis of proteins is involved.[11, 12]

Nitric oxide in the cardiovascular system in septic shock

The physiological importance of nitric oxide in the regulation of the vascular system is well established. Nitric oxide is synthesized from L-arginine by the action of nitric oxide synthase (NOS).[13] There are currently known to be three distinct isoforms: neuronal NOS (nNOS) also known as type I, inducible NOS (iNOS) or type II NOS and endothelial constitutive NOS (ecNOS) or type III NOS. The nNOS and ecNOS isoforms are constitutively expressed but require stimulation of the calmodulin–calcium pathway for enzyme activation, through increased intracellular calcium, by substances such as bradykinin and acetylcholine. The synthesis and release of nitric oxide by the constitutive enzymes is rapid and independent of *de novo* protein synthesis. In contrast, iNOS expression relies on stimulation by cytokines or endotoxin and synthesis of the iNOS protein, which takes several hours. Nitric oxide is a free radical (it has an unpaired electron) and is therefore highly reactive. Nitric oxide activates soluble guanylate cyclase to catalyse the formation of cyclic guanosine 5′ phosphate (cGMP). This results in changes in intracellular calcium concentrations and relaxation of smooth muscle.

Perfusion of rat hearts or isolated cardiac myocytes with nitric oxide donors causes depressed contractility, associated with the release of cGMP.[14] This and other studies indicate that, in addition to its role in regulation of vascular tone, nitric oxide and cGMP have profound regulatory effects on cardiac contractility. Circulating metabolites of nitric oxide, NOS enzyme activity and cGMP are increased during sepsis.[15–17]

Experimental evidence showed that the myocardial depressive effect of TNFα in rat myocytes *in vitro* could be obliterated by inhibitors of nitric oxide formation such as L-NMMA or methylene blue.[18, 19] Conversely, the addition of the substrate for NOS, L-arginine, re-established myocardial depression.[20] These data indicated that the myocardial depression is mediated at a subcellular level through production of nitric oxide, mediated via generation of cGMP, likely to be via up-regulation of type II NOS (inducible isoform). Clearly this involves *de novo* protein synthesis, and early myocardial effects cannot be explained, since induction of type II NOS takes several hours. It is likely therefore that the process involves both type II and type I NOS (constitutive).

However, the story is not simple. In addition to nitric oxide we believe there is also a second discrete cardiodepressant mechanism concomitantly present. Exposure of rat myocytes to TNFα results in early defective contractile responses to adrenaline (epinephrine) or isoproterenol, which cannot be corrected.[21, 22] The defect is associated with TNFα-mediated reductions in catecholamine stimulated cyclic adenosine 5′ monophosphate (cAMP) release. Later onset cytokine-mediated cardiac myocyte depression has also demonstrated defects of catecholamine-stimulated contractility and cAMP generation.[23] This late adrenergic signal transduction defect was at least partially related to myocardial induction of type II NOS. Interestingly, induction of type II NOS alone was not sufficient to cause contractile hyporesponsiveness in this model. These data suggest that TNFα, and possibly other cytokines implicated in septic shock, exerts its effects by an early mechanism that is nitric oxide-dependent but adrenoreceptor-independent, coupled with a nitric oxide independent defect of β-adrenergic signal transduction. Late myocardial depression, however, seemed to involve a type II NOS-dependent defect of β-adrenergic signal transduction.

As a general concept, understanding the subcellular physiological mechanisms involved in septic shock results in better clinical management of patients. For example, the results of experiments involving adrenaline (epinephrine) can be taken into the treatment arena. In the *in vitro* study adrenaline (epinephrine)-mediated contractile dysfunction was not reversible, because of decreased cAMP as described above. Phosphodiesterases are the enzymes responsible for the breakdown of cAMP and cGMP, such that phosphodiesterase inhibitors maintain cAMP/cGMP levels. If in the clinical setting a phosphodiesterase inhibitor, such as amiodarone, is given, it is possible to override the abnormality impressively and correct the defect in myocyte contractility.

Nitric oxide and the vasculature

There is much data to suggest that excessive nitric oxide release is responsible for the decreased systemic vascular resistance, vasodilatation, and low blood pressure seen in patients with septic shock. Persistent vasodilatation characteristic of septic shock may result from overproduction of nitric oxide and can lead to hypotension that is refractory to vasopressors and may result in death. To evaluate the significance of cytokine-inducible nitric oxide synthase, type II NOS, in the pathogenesis of sepsis, Hollenberg *et al.*[24] used a clinically relevant mouse model of sepsis and compared mortality and microvascular reactivity in wild-type mice and so called 'knock-out' mice, which lacked the gene for the type II NOS enzyme. Mice were made septic by caecal ligation and puncture, fluid-resuscitated, and given antibiotics. Microvascular vasoconstriction in response to topical noradrenaline (norepinephrine) was measured in cremasteric arterioles using videomicroscopy. Mortality at 48 hours was significantly lower in septic knock-out mice (45%) than in wild-type mice (76%). Vasoconstrictive responses to noradrenaline (norepinephrine) were significantly better in septic-type II NOS knock-out mice than in wild-type septic mice. This elegant study showed that microvascular catecholamine responsiveness and survival were improved in mice lacking the gene for type II NOS in a clinically relevant model of sepsis, suggesting that type II NOS plays an important, but not an exclusive, role in refractory vasodilatation in patients with septic shock.

Inhibition of nitric oxide in septic shock

In animal models of sepsis, intravenous administration of low doses of the nitric oxide inhibitor, the arginine analogue, L-N^G-monomethylarginine (L-NMMA), prevents the fall in blood pressure after endotoxin administration and prevents mortality. High doses of L-NMMA, however, cause an acute increase in blood pressure followed by a rapid fall and increased mortality.[25] The increased mortality is accompanied by increased tissue damage suggesting both beneficial and detrimental effects of nitric oxide in endotoxic shock.[25-27] This can be explained by considering the role of constitutively formed nitric oxide (via type II NOS) in the physiological control of blood pressure. Nitric oxide from type III NOS provides normal vasodilator tone and its inhibition raises blood pressure and reduces blood flow. High doses of L-NMMA will inhibit this in addition to type II-mediated nitric oxide synthesis. The adverse effect of high doses of L-NMMA in endotoxin-treated animals can be prevented if a nitrovasodilator is given to replace lost constitutive nitric oxide-mediated vasodilator tone.[28]

L-NMMA has also been given to patients with septic shock. Initial anecdotal case reports appeared promising, and a phase II trial showed increased blood pressure, decreased circulating nitrite/nitrate concentrations, and resulted in significantly more patients in whom shock resolved within 72 hours.[29] However, a subsequent phase III trial designed to investigate the effect of L-NMMA on mortality was prematurely stopped because of safety concerns.

Conclusion

It is clear that much of the pathophysiology of sepsis and the cardiovascular system remain incompletely understood. As the complicated mechanisms involved become clearer, physicians will be in a better position in terms of treating patients, and soon we may be able to offer effective specific treatment for this very devastating disease.

References

1   Wilson F. Surgical intensive care units. In: Parrillo JE, Ayres SM, eds. *Major Issues in Critical Care Medicine*. Baltimore: Williams & Wilkins, 1984.

2   Parker MM, Parrillo JE, Septic shock. Hemodynamics and pathogenesis. *J Am Med Assoc* 1983;**250**:3324–7.

3   Parrillo JE. Septic shock in humans: advances in the understanding of pathogenesis, cardiovascular dysfunction and therapy. *Ann Intern Med* 1990;**113**:227–42.3

4   Parker MM, Shelhamer JH, Natanson C, Alling DW, Parrillo JE. Serial cardiovascular variables in survivors and non-survivors of human septic shock: heart rate as an early predictor of prognosis. *Crit Care Med* 1987;**15**:923–9.

5   Parker MM, Suffredini AF, Natanson C, Ognibene FP, Shelhamer JH, Parrillo JE. Responses of left ventricular function in survivors and non-survivors in septic shock. *J Crit Care* 1989;**4**:19–25.

6   Danner RL, Elin RJ, Hoseini JM, *et al.* Endotoxin determinations in 100 patients with septic shock. *Clin Res* 1988;**36**:453A (abstract).

7   Suffredini AF, Fromm RE, Parker MM, *et al.* The cardiovascular response of normal humans to the administration of endotoxin. *NEJM* 1989;**321**:280–7.

8   Natanson C, Danner RL, Elin RJ, *et al.* The role of endotoxemia in cardiovascular dysfunction and mortality. *Escherichia coli* and *Staphylococcus aureus* challenges in a canine model of human septic shock. *J Clin Invest* 1989;**83**:243–51.

9   Parrillo JE, Burch C, Shelhamer JH, Parker MM, Natanson C, Schuette W. A circulating myocardial depressant substance in humans with septic shock. Septic shock patients with a reduced ejection fraction have a circulating factor that depresses *in vitro* myocardial cell performance. *J Clin Invest* 1985;**76**:1539–53.

10 Kumar A, Thota V, Dee L, Olson J, Uretz E, Parrillo J. Tumor necrosis factor α and interleukin 1β are responsible for *in vitro* myocardial cell depression induced by human septic shock serum. *J Exp Med* 1996;**183**:949–58.

11 Gulick T, Chung MK, Pieper SJ, Lange LG, Schreiner GF. Interleukin-1 and tumor necrosis factor inhibit cardiac myocyte adrenergic responsiveness. *Proc Natl Acad Sci* 1989;**86**:6753–7.

12 DeMeules JE, Pigula FA, Mueller M, Raymond SJ, Gamelli RL. Tumor necrosis factor and cardiac function. *J Trauma* 1992;**32**:686–92.

13 Galley HF, Webster NR. Nitric oxide in a nutshell: genetics, physiology and pathology. *Curr Anaesth Crit Care* 1998;**9**:209–13.

14 Wahler GM, Dollinger SJ. Nitric oxide donor SIN-1 inhibits mammalian cardiac calcium current through cGMP-dependant protein kinase. *Am J Physiol* 1995;**268** to replace lost constitutive nitric oxide-mediated vasodilator tone C45–54.

15 Ochoa JB, Udekwu AO, Billiar TR, *et al.* Nitrogen oxide levels in patients after trauma and during sepsis. *Ann Surg* 1991;**214**:621–6.

16 Goode HF, Howdle PD, Walker BE, Webster NR. Nitric oxide synthase activity is increased in patients with sepsis syndrome. *Clin Sci* 1995;**88**:131–3.

17 Rosenberg RB, Broner CW, O'Dorisio MS. Modulation of cyclic guanosine monophosphate production during *Escherichia coli* septic shock. *Biochem Med Metab Biol* 1994;**51**:149–55.

18 Schneider F, Lutun P, Hasselmann M, Stoclet JC, Tempe JD. Methylene blue increases systemic vascular resistance in human septic shock. Preliminary observations. *Intens Care Med* 1992;**18**:309–11.

19 Petros A, Lamb G, Leone A, Moncada S, Bennett D, Vallance P. Effects of a

nitric oxide synthase inhibitor in humans with septic shock. *Cardiovasc Res* 1994;**28**:34–9.

20 Kumar A, Kosuri R, Thota V, *et al*. Nitric oxide and cGMP generation mediates human septic shock serum-induced *in vitro* cardiomyocyte depression. *Chest* 1993;**104**:12S (abstract).

21 Kumar A, Thota V, Kosuri R, *et al*. Tumor necrosis factor impairs epinephrine-stimulated cardiomyocyte contractility and cyclic AMP production via a nitric oxide-independent mechanism. *Crit Care Med* 1996;**23**:A148 (abstract).

22 Kumar A, Brar R, Sun E, Olson J, Parrillo JE. Tumor necrosis factor (TNF) impairs isoproterenol stimulated cardiac myocyte contractility and cyclic AMP production via a nitric oxide independent mechanism. *Crit Care Med* 1996;**24**:A95 (abstract).

23 Chung MK, Gulick TS, Rotondo RE, Schreiner GF, Lange LG. Mechanism of cytokine inhibition of beta-adrenergic agonist stimulation of cyclic AMP in rat cardiac myocytes: impairment of signal transduction. *Circ Res* **67**:753–63.

24 Hollenberg SM, Broussard M, Osman J, Parrillo JE. Increased microvascular reactivity and improved mortality in septic mice lacking inducible nitric oxide synthase. *Circ Res* 2000;**86**:774–9.

25 Nava E, Palmer RMJ, Moncada S. Inhibition of nitric oxide synthesis in septic shock: how much is beneficial? *Lancet* 1991;**2**:1555–7.

26 Thiemermann C, Vane J. Inhibition of nitric oxide synthesis reduces the hypotension induced by bacterial lipopolysaccharides in the rat *in vivo*. *Eur J Pharmacol* 1990;**182**:591–5.

27 Billiar TR, Curran RD, Harbrecht BG, Stuehr DJ, Demetris AJ, Simmons RL. Modulation of nitrogen oxide synthesis in vivo: NG-monomethyl-L-arginine inhibits endotoxin-induced nitrate/nitrite biosynthesis while promoting hepatic damage. *J Leukocyte Biol* 1990;**48**:565–9.

28 Wright CE, Rees DD, Moncada S. Protective and pathological roles of nitric oxide in endotoxin shock. *Cardiovasc Res* 1992;**26**:48–57.

29 Anzueto A, Beale R, Holzapfel L, Arneson C, Grover R. Multicentre placebo controlled double blind study of the nitric oxide synthase inhibitor 546C88 in patients with septic shock: effect on resolution of shock and survival. *Intensive Care Med* 1997;**23**(Suppl. 1): S57 (abstract).

Index

Please note: page numbers in **bold** type refer to figures, and those in *italics* refer to tables or boxed material.

INDEX